The Passionate Mind

a manual for living creatively with one's self

Joel Kramer

Edited by Jules Kanarek

Drawings by Dora Cornwall

North Atlantic Books
Berkeley, California

D1057335

The Passionate Mind

Copyright © 1974, 1983 by Joel Kramer. No portion of this book, except for brief review, may be reproduced, stored in a retrieval system, or transmitted, in any form or by any means, electronic, mechanical, photocopying, recording or otherwise without the written permission of the publisher. For information contact the publisher.

Published by
North Atlantic Books
P.O. Box 12327
Berkeley, California 94712

Cover design by Paula Morrison

The Passionate Mind is sponsored by the Society for the Study of Native Arts and Sciences, a nonprofit educational corporation whose goals are to develop an educational and crosscultural perspective linking various scientific, social, and artistic fields; to nurture a holistic view of arts, sciences, humanities, and healing; and to publish and distribute literature on the relationship of mind, body, and nature.

Library of Congress Cataloging-in-Publication Data

Kramer, Joel, 1937–
    The passionate mind,
      1. Self-perception.   2. Thought and thinking.   3. Meditation
    4. Emotions. I. Title
    BF697.K68   131'.32   74–6047
    ISBN 0-938190-12-1

        8 9 10 11 12 / 02 01 00 99 98 97

FOREWORD

Editing these lectures by Joel Kramer has been a stimulating and enlightening experience. The editing of a series of lectures can be a tedious process since one generally has to reread the same passages over and over again. But each time I reread a passage from these lectures, invariably, it felt new and fresh and seemed to kindle some new spark of understanding, some new flicker of awareness.

For those interested in encountering a different prospectus on the game of life, this book may have a profound effect. It delves deep into areas our conditioned minds are reluctant to probe. It goes beyond the world of ideas, beliefs, and images in which each of us personally lives to reveal the obvious, the "what is" that is constantly dangling before our very eyes, but which most of us could spend an entire lifetime not seeing.

Thousands of books have been written about the world around us. This book explores the world within. It takes the reader on an exciting adventure into the unknown—himself. It presents a new way of seeing, a new understanding of being. The trip may not be pleasant at times, but it's always revealing.

The validity of Joel Kramer's presentation must be judged by each reader individually. Hopefully, it will encourage a new way of seeing so that readers can continue this exciting adventure after they've reached the final page.

—Jules Kanarek

PREFACE

This book represents years of talking with people about the fundamental problems of living. It is a collection of transcribed and edited lectures. It is also an expression of my own inner inquiry.

Stylistically there may appear to be a terseness and austerity that makes more of a demand on the reader than is ordinarily the case. The conversational mode of presentation may initially take a getting used to. The difficulty is that with words I am attempting to communicate aspects of being that are fundamentally nonverbal. The precision of the language was my main concern. While the presentation may at first appear unusual, I feel it contains a directness and simplicity that can be seen by any human being really interested in exploring the nature of him or herself.

—Joel Kramer

TABLE OF CONTENTS

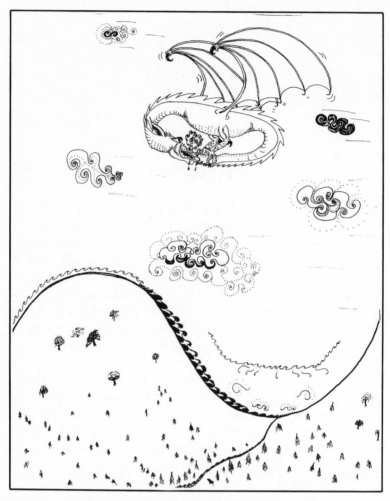

Memry the Dragon is always gnawing his Self

INTRODUCTION TO THE ILLUSTRATIONS

In reading each section of Joel's talks an image came forth that for me embodied the chapter. Historically the dragon has been a symbol in the West of fear and in the East of knowledge. Fear and knowledge are the stuff of memory . . . and so the central figure of the drawings is a dragon I call Memry.

—Dora Cornwall

INTRODUCTION

What we are going to be doing in these talks, which are ideally not monologues at all, but discussions, dialogues between you and me, is to examine fundamentally the nature of what it is to be a human being. In order to do this, it is necessary for us to actually look at ourselves as we are. That's not such an easy thing to do because we have all kinds of ideas about what an individual ought to be or should be; all kinds of desires as to what we want to be. This clouds our vision so that it becomes very difficult for us to see ourselves as we are. It's not possible to see clearly anything at all, until we come into contact with ourselves.

All of the things that go under the name of Yoga, or meditational pursuits, or high energy games, or spiritual interests have one thing in common. They all have as a focus a quieting of mind, a quieting of thought, a quieting of the whole intellectual, computerlike process. Of course, the most natural question that one might ask oneself is "Why do this, why do this at all?" We have been conditioned with thought; our very educational system trains us to have very active, very busy, very comparing and competitive minds. And, of course, the sharper, the cleverer, the better we are in our intellectual processes, the more we are rewarded by society and the world; we reap the goods and the rewards that the world gives us for our cleverness. Yet the whole nature of meditation directs itself to quieting this whole process—to there being a silence in oneself.

The real question is "Why? Why do this?" In order to see why it might be interesting for there to be a quietness of thought, it is necessary to look at what thought is all about. In order to see why meditation as a way of living might be extraordinary, it is necessary

1

to see the whole nature of thought. That is what we are going to be doing in the time we spend together.

In order to do this it is vital that we look at ourselves. If I am just another authority for you, then you aren't going to look at yourselves. There are many authorities in the world. You go to one person and he says "Do this," and you go to another and he says "Do that," and a third says "Don't do anything those people told you, only I know what's right, so do what I say"; and this is endless. I go from one authority to another and they tell me to listen to them. What am I to do? I go here and I'm told to do this. I go there and I'm told to do that. I go somewhere else and I'm told to do something else. What am I to do? So I shop around until I find someone who tells me what I want to hear and I obey him. This is what is ordinarily called learning or growth, which, of course, is not learning at all.

What we are going to be doing together is to do away with authority totally, so that we need no one, and then you actually can become an authority for yourself—a light for yourself. Of course, in order to do this you must come to terms with yourself. You must see yourself, and to do this, you must look. That is hopefully what we are going to do together—look at ourselves.

These words are at best a mirror—a mirror for you to see yourself in. The words themselves are not what they purport to represent. Insofar as they are words they are always inadequate, always an abstraction. The nature of language is such that it makes real communication very difficult indeed. Take any word. Take a common noun like *cat*. You know that the word itself is an abstraction and by that I mean something quite simple. Philosophically, to abstract means to fail to take account of. So that if I say "Here is a cat," I have failed to take account of whether it is a black cat or white, male or female, young or old, brown-eyed or blue-eyed, with short hair or long hair, or an infinite number of actual attributes— its relation to the room, its relation to me, its temperament, etc. If I were trying with symbols to describe totally the livingness of this cat, to hold it in words, I would have to express myself indefinitely, the living thing is not the word. A living thing is always moving, always changing. If I were to string an infinite number of adjectives before the noun *cat* (which, of course, is not possible), I still would just have words, not a living cat. Yet we are dealing with words here, and through words we are trying to communicate. What this person is talking about is something that fundamentally cannot be communicated by words. However, we are going to be using words in speaking with each other. So it is with this in mind that we should be aware that the word is not the thing. It is possible, if we are very careful, very intelligent, to see the limitation of the symbolic-verbal approach. To see this is to get in touch with the nature and limitations of thought, since thought operates with symbols.

Thought tells itself it is limitless, that it can handle all problems. All that is needed is the proper structure, formula or system. There are problems the very nature of which thought is not equipped to handle. We will be examining problems that can only be approached by an intelligence not bound by thought.

Meditation has to do with the quieting of the computer, the quieting of the intellectual, verbal process. Yet a mind that is trying to quiet itself to achieve this quietness, is a very active, very busy mind. We are also going to examine whether or not thought can quiet itself. This is one of the problems or paradoxes of meditation.

One of the problems in these discussions is that it is extremely difficult to listen, whether it be to this person or to anyone else. Ordinarily what we do when we think we are listening is to take in the words, translate them into something that we know or are familiar with, and then agree or disagree. If the words fit our structures, our beliefs, the things we are comfortable with, the things we know, then the speaker is a wise man and we agree. If the words do not please us, do not fit our structures and beliefs, do not give us pleasure, then the speaker is not a wise man and we disagree. That's what most of us do, and call it listening. But if we are either agreeing or disagreeing, then we're not listening, for to listen there must be an openness, an innocence, a putting away of the old ideas, so that possibly the fresh can come in. If you are busily involved in either agreeing or disagreeing (and you can watch yourself do this as you listen), then what you are doing is not listening at all, and the new, which is the fount of growth and learning, does not come in. I think it will be the case, for many of us, that what we are going to talk about, and the way we are going to do this, will be new. This person is not interested at all in having you agree with him. He is interested in having you look at yourself so perhaps the words can be a mirror for you to see yourself in. To agree is totally meaningless.

I am interested in having you listen so that perhaps you can decide for yourself whether what is being said is true or not true for you. But you can only do this if you are listening, which involves an openness, an innocence, and a *passionate mind.* Real passion occurs only when there is a giving up of oneself, an abandonment. Only in passion is there a quality of attention fundamental to learning. You really have to care about seeing (in this case it is seeing yourself) and this never involves agreement or disagreement. For as soon as you say "I know," then growth stops.

There's another problem in communication. In order for it to occur, there must be a sense of communion, a sense of touch, a sense of being together and exploring things together. Communication never occurs when there's either dominance or submission. The very nature of dominance and submission destroys the energy of communication. Why do I dominate you or try to? I do it to get you to do what I want, or to make myself feel good, or to feel superior, to control you for my own wants. Why do I submit to you? I submit only if you have something I want. Perhaps I submit out of fear, which means there are experiences or other "things" I want from you or don't want from you; I submit in order to control you for my own wants.

If you examine the nature of dominance and submission carefully, you will find that they are not opposites, but rather the same thing in different guises. Both are used in order to control. Real communication, which is not merely the superficial intellectual understanding of words, occurs only when there's a sense of equality. Only when there is this sense of equality can we explore with our total being the deeper questions that display themselves in living. Dominance or submission, which is either being an authority or obeying one, cuts off learning.

Most of us are secondhand human beings. What we are, what we believe, the way we move through the world, are all secondhand, gathered from books and other authorities, from our conditioning, from experiences handed to us. So that actually we are just recreating the past over and over again which is never new, never fresh. It doesn't matter what somebody else says, or what the great or wise say. We don't know that they're great or wise; we imagine they are, somebody has told us, or we read a book and the book says they are. To be concerned with such matters is not to be looking at oneself.

It's difficult to do away with all authority because it puts one in a rather frightening place. There is nothing to hold on to. Yet real learning, which is not merely the accumulation of knowledge, which has nothing at all to do with the mechanical repetition of what we call knowledge, real learning never occurs unless we do away with authority.

We are going to examine many of the basic problems of living—many of the fundamental problems of being a human being in the world today. Contrary to much that we read or hear, meditation is not a removal from the world. Meditation is being in the world in a very intimate way. We are going to examine what it is to be a human being in the world today. To do this, we are going to look at many of the so-called perennial problems of man: the problems of pleasure and pain, the problems of belief and freedom, sorrow, fear and desire, conflict, time and death, love, sexuality. *We* are the world, and these problems as they express themselves in the world also express themselves in us. In order to solve the world's problems, it's essential to solve problems in ourselves—the problems of day-to-day living.

One might ask, "Why bother to do this at all?" The tremendous push that most of us are feeling because of the pressures of the times is very demanding. Is not this whole involvement with awareness a very self-centered activity, a withdrawing into oneself? Why be so self-centered? The world and society are breaking down. The very planet that we are living on is becoming uninhabitable. The ecological problems, the problem of overpopulation in the cities, the problem of violence, poverty, war, of sorrow of one sort or another— the extraordinary problems of living in the world today, I am sure are obvious to each and every one of you. Is there anything meaningful in all this self-inquiry to answer these problems?

All of the problems of the world are created by human beings, and problems do not change until human beings do. It is only if there is real change in human beings that there will ever be an answer to these problems, because these problems have been gathering over the centuries and they now seem to be coming to a head. When we look at the nature of evolution, I think we will find that what we are involved in has to do with the basic problem of survival, as to whether or not we are going to be able to live on this world, which means living with one another. The old order isn't working, the old ways are breaking down and there isn't anything viable that is coming to the fore. In these days there are many experiments with so-called new ways of living. Still solutions to these problems do not seem to be coming. The reason is that the problems are simply the problems of being a human being, and unless there is a real change in the very structure of the mind and heart of human beings, there never is any real change at all. The external problems are just a manifestation of the internal. The problems of the world are created by people and they are expressions of people. The greed of the world is the expression of my greed. The violence of the world is the expression of my violence. And it doesn't change unless I do. The question is: Is it possible for an ordinary human being, a human being like you and me, to come to terms with himself so that the human being can individually, personally (because it is all very personal), meet the challenges of living in these extraordinarily turbulent times?

CHAPTER 1

BELIEF

What we believe determines much of what we think and do: the way
we move, the way we respond to people, how we think of ourselves,
how we see the world in general. But what does it mean to believe in
anything—a man, a philosophy, a system of ideas, a religion, an
economic system? Let's not ask if a belief is right or wrong, good or
bad, life-furthering or destroying, but rather just what it means to
be in a state of belief. I would like for us to look at the whole structure of belief: It is a doorway into the nature of thought.

I have a belief about anything. How does this affect the whole
internal structure of my awareness? Exactly what does it mean to be
in a state of belief? Let's look at it personally, each of us.

For a human being to have a belief, to be in a state of belief, there
is one thing that is quite obvious. To be in a state of belief means
there is no firsthand personal knowledge. If one is in a state of
intimate, direct understanding then there is no belief. I think we will
be able to look—inwardly look—and see the difference so that one
can tell for oneself whether one is actually in a state of belief or not.

To believe anything at all is to be in a state of violence—external
and internal violence. Let us see the way this works.

As one moves through the world one sees there are many beliefs
which are always jockeying with one another, always vying for our
minds. If you have a belief about anything and that belief is attacked
by another belief—another system of thought, philosophy, religion,
another "ism"—what do you do? You automatically defend it, don't
you? The thing to do is look at the way you work. Whether you
defend it verbally to the other person or go away and defend it

7

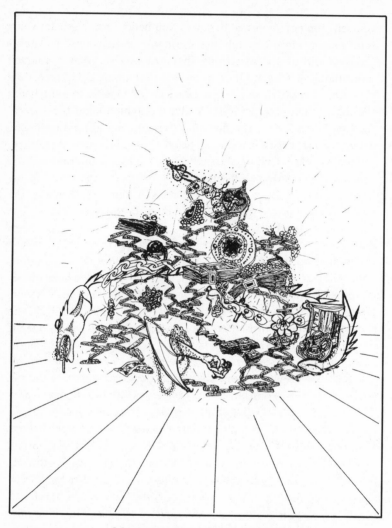

Memry's security buries his Self

silently to yourself doesn't matter—you're still defending it. It's in the psychological structure of belief to automatically defend itself when attacked.

Is a defense any different from attack? To be defending a belief is to be attacking somebody else's. In this whole process of belief there is always defense and attack—always. You can observe this in yourself. I'm not interested in having you believe me, see it for yourself. As you move through the world in relationships, inevitably someone will attack something that you believe. Watch yourself immediately defend it. It is from this that there is violence, real violence, internal violence. You can feel the tension in your body: the constrictions happen in the body, the tightening of the viscera, the tone of the voice, the flow of adrenalin, the aggression in the defense. So that to be in a state of belief is to be in a state of violence, internal violence. And of course the violence that is internal and the violence that is external are not different. I make the world in my image, and if there is internal violence, it expresses itself in the world. All one has to do is to look around in the world today. The expression is quite obvious.

However, if I personally, firsthand know anything at all, if the understanding, which is much more than intellectual recognition, is internal, if it is not secondhand, then there is a whole different process involved. If somebody were to tell me the earth is flat, I might initially respond by saying that it is really round. If he should continue to insist that it's flat, I would begin to wonder if this man is putting me on, or if he's operating with some mental quirk, or if he's a little insane, or whatever. You can observe in yourself that there isn't the inward psychological push to defend yourself. This is something that you know. Of course, it is possible that the earth being round is a deep-seated belief gained secondhand through books or through common knowledge. It it is, somewhere you will find a defense mechanism come into play. Some beliefs are so highly conditioned, so ingrained, it may appear there is no defense taking place. In fact, should one believe that beliefs are violent, there may be effort applied not to defend one's beliefs, to prove to oneself that they are not beliefs at all. But the physiology does not easily fool itself. Tensions, glandular changes, the effort itself, all are clues.

When you have internal understanding that is not based upon what somebody else says, then there isn't the necessity, the internal psychological push to defend yourself. To identify your beliefs, you must watch yourself closely because defense is automatic. As soon as you're attacked you defend, either overtly by punching someone in the nose (or wanting to), or verbally by attacking the person, or quietly to yourself—all such responses are violent. You can observe this in little things, and big ones, as you move through the world: in the ways you operate with your friends, with your family, in any relationship.

Do you know that all the violence in the world is done in the name of belief—every last bit of it? It's all done in the name of truth and beauty and goodness and righteousness and all of these very, very highsounding things. To see how this works in oneself is essential for awareness. Of course, to see it is not necessarily to make it go away. I see beliefs and I say I must make them go away because I'm a violent person and I want to be a nonviolent person. Having beliefs makes me violent, so I don't want beliefs. I want them to go away and I want to become nonviolent. But that's another belief: the belief that I should be nonviolent. To try to make beliefs go away is, again, to be avoiding yourself or what you are on the basis of another belief—hence more violence.

Here is a man telling you that to be in a state of belief is violent and if you believe it and try to make your beliefs go away, you're just getting involved in it again. So what do you do? That is one of the questions we will look at here. The question of what is one to do. Look, I see I have beliefs. I see that they create violence. I see that any effort I make to change this I do out of another belief—for example, that I be nonviolent. I see how this also creates more violence. What to do?

Do I replace my beliefs with another belief I can tolerate? When I see the whole structure of belief, it's not a question of which beliefs I can tolerate, because by their very nature the beliefs that I have inculcated into me are the ones I can tolerate. I tend to think in terms of good beliefs and bad beliefs: the beliefs that further me and the ones that don't. But we're not looking at that, we're looking at the structure of belief, any belief. To see any belief at all is to see how it brings forth violence—is violence. It doesn't matter what the nature of it is. For example, I may believe that a human being should be nonviolent. That is a *good* belief, a life-furthering belief. Yet any belief, even a belief in nonviolence, only perpetuates the very thing I'm trying to do away with—violence. In some places people don't kill rats because belief in nonviolence is a way of living. In the guise of worshipping the sanctity of all life, rats are not killed and are left free to roam the streets and eat children—which actually happens. So, in the name of nonviolence, greater violence is committed, which is the way of any belief.

It's important to see the structure of belief, not specific beliefs, but any belief. How do you get your beliefs? They are conditioned into you. There are hopes, fears, and desires. What gives you pleasure you tend to move toward; what you find unpleasant you tend to move away from. So you attempt to incorporate structures that make you feel good and do away with structures that don't. I'm not saying you should or should not do this; this person is not interested in what one should or should not do. What we are looking at is what is, and how it works. To see how beliefs work, even beliefs that presumably make me feel better, is to see violence in them and how they are deadening things, how they turn me off from seeing the world and living in it. If I have a belief about anything, it means I have cut off inquiry. Instead of looking, I believe, and that's a deadening, habitual thing. It stiffens me and makes me tired. To see this—really to see it—brings forth movement. Later, we'll look at the nature of this movement.

The nature of belief is a fundamental consideration. What we're discussing here is a way of looking at what is—not what I want to be, not what others tell me should or should not be, or what authorities say—but a way of looking at what is.

If I look only at what I want to see, then I don't look at all. If I want to understand anything—a flower, a child, anything—then I must observe it, I must watch it carefully. If I'm involved in trying to make it something other than what it is, if I'm involved in trying to change it, trying to improve it, I'm no longer watching it. I am now, through effort, trying to manipulate, and if I do that I'm no longer seeing the reality of the thing, whatever that thing is. This is also true of oneself. If you really want to understand what you are and how you work, you must watch yourself. Trying to become something better or different removes you from the watching. Yet the reality of it is I do want to become better; I am interested in changing, being higher, more enlightened, more spiritual, fulfilled, realized. So one of the things that I am is a being always trying to change itself. But I can watch that and see just what it means to be always involved in attempting to change myself—which is not trying to change the fact that I'm trying to change myself. I can observe that the effort involved in attempting to change comes from ideas that I should be different, and that these ideas are beliefs conditioned into me, so that any change that involves effort comes from belief, which is violence. If I watch this reality of myself always wanting to be something other than what I am, I can begin to see the movement of that which is me. All of this lives in thought. What it is saying is that I should be better. Is it not thought that is saying this? What is trying to change me? Is it not thought, based on memory that is always trying to make me into something other than what I am? That is one of the things we will look at very deeply.

To see the entire structure of belief is to get in touch with a whole way of looking that has to do with seeing what is, for it is seeing what is that is itself living awareness. Awareness is the direct relationship with what is.

Question. Are you telling us what you know?
Answer. I'm not telling you anything. I'm talking to you about a way of looking at yourself. About a way of looking. It's not mine; it's not a possession or an invention. It's just there. All one has to do is look. You can look at the structure of belief, and one only does this in day-to-day living. You can walk down the street and observe how you operate with people. When a belief of yours is attacked, you can watch how you respond, because only then will you find out. The reality of it is that most of us have beliefs, innumerable beliefs, big and little about this and that, and they are all functions of habit, all very deadening things, very dull things. To see this you must look at them. Nobody can do it for you.

Question. Are you saying that if you don't like what you see and make an effort to change, you are causing violence? If so, how else can change occur?
Answer. In the first place, to say that you don't like what you see automatically means you are not seeing. You are judging, placing a value. This is thought or the mind saying what ought to be, and ought-to-be's are just beliefs, therefore there is no seeing. How does change occur? Where does help come from? Help only comes

from one place—yourself. One can observe that one lives in conflict. I observe my beliefs. I observe the fact that I don't like them and want them to go away. I observe the fact that the very process of doing this creates conflict. Ordinarily when I look, I don't look in order to see. I look in order to change. I look with an eye towards making myself better or something else. Why we want to change is one of the things we will look at. We have an idea that there is a way to be that is different from the way we are. Just what the idea is, is an always nebulous changing thing, and we are continually hungering after something else. Looking at yourself is not analysis, not introspection. We have an idea that looking is a going over and analyzing and tearing apart of something that has happened in the past. It's not that at all; looking is something quite different. If there is conflict, there is conflict; the more I try to make conflict go away, the more conflict I create. Conflict as we'll see later is quite involved with belief.

Chapter 2

PLEASURE

What are we searching for? We are all looking for something, aren't we? What is it that one seeks? What are we after? There are many names for people's searching; self-realization, actuality, enlightenment, spirituality, higher levels of consciousness, freedom, peace, nirvana, samadi. And we shouldn't omit health, love, strength, so many things that people seek. If we look beyond the words, beyond all of these names, I think one will find that what we are really looking for is something called *pleasure*. We want to feel good, to feel better and better. So we continually seek a state of feeling better.

In seeking anything at all, you can only seek the known; you can't seek the unknown. Suppose I were to tell you to go ahead and look for something that was totally out of your ken, something completely out of your experience. How would you go about finding it? Where would you look? How would you know when you found it? You would only know if you recognize it. You only recognize something if you already know it. You can only seek what you know.

Actually, what we are seeking are things we hold in memory; experiences we now judge to be pleasurable or sublime, or whatever we call it. Five minutes ago, or last year, twenty years ago, I had an extraordinary experience which, of course, now lives in memory. That experience, whether it be the initial blush of young love or something that happened under a drug or an infantile feeling of security that sometimes occurs in the very young—whatever it was, it has been cherished over the years. When I'm feeling bad I think of it, it warms me, and I say, "Wouldn't it be nice if I could be that way

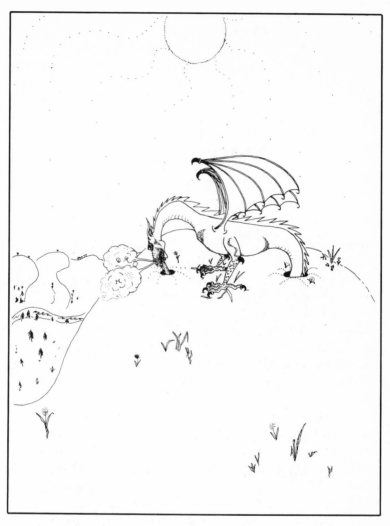

Memry catches himself

all of the time, or at least more than I now am?" When we seek, is it not this that we seek—a repetition or intensification of the known? You can only seek something that has happened. You cannot seek the new because it's unknown; you can seek only the old. You may think that you're seeking something new. You're tired of your old life, bored with it, you want something different. People tell you of wonderful states of being. Books entice you with their mysteries and promises of delights beyond comprehension. You say to yourself, "That's for me." Then you search for the key to unlock the door to all of these goodies. What are these "goodies"? Do you not simply translate all of these ideas into other words or images that come from your experience? Please look in yourself and see if this is so. Searching for the "unknown" is simply seeking ideas. Ideas are nothing but the creation of thought—which is always old. Thoughts can rearrange themselves to appear new, yet these products of imagination are not really new. They are simply the old in disguise. It is also very easy to get wrapped up in the pleasures of search itself. Let's look at what we are seeking, which goes under many names, but is adequately described as "pleasure." To look at pleasure and see how it works is an inroad to the nature of thought.

It's early in the morning and I'm walking down the beach. There isn't a soul in sight. I am alone. The sun is rising over the mountains, there's a burst of sunlight over the water. For a moment (it doesn't matter if the moment is a second or half an hour), the gap, the space between the experiencer and the experience is not there. There is no separation; there is just the experience. There is just the relationship of the seer and the seen; it is one thing. Here and there, in living, it is probable that most of us have had a moment of this sort. It is in such moments that it's possible to see the nature of pleasure.

What usually happens first? What do you first become aware of at such times? Does not the evaluative process come in? You say, "This is beautiful, this is lovely, this is extraordinary"—whatever it is that you say. Then perhaps you wonder how you can get back and do it again. How can you do it a lot, or tomorrow, or next year, or five years from now? Isn't this the kind of thing that happens? It is here that one begins to find out the nature of pleasure. The experience of that moment, that timelessness, was just what it was—it is only after it happens that you say it is good, I like it. You try to repeat it or you look for it again. Actually, pleasure does not live in the moment itself; pleasure lives only in the memory of the moment as you evaluate it, as you call it good and seek its repetition. The experience may have had an extraordinary quality, an energy. But that is gone as soon as evaluation comes in. There is an evaluator, an experiencer who is (actually was) having an experience, which means there is separation. As soon as you're aware you're having an experience, it's gone, isn't it? The evaluator and the evaluation are not separate. When the evaluation occurs the evaluator is the evaluation, and that is what's going on, not the experience that is being evaluated. The experience now lives only in memory.

Can you see how this works for you, not the words, but the actuality of what it means to be evaluating? Not whether I should or should not be evaluating (judging, which is, of course, just evaluation again), but how evaluation works in living. Strong experiences leave a residue in thought and in the tissue—the cells themselves. I bask in the memory of it; it warms me. Here is where pleasure lies: in the memory, not in the experience itself. The experience simply is. Pleasure comes in after the fact. Watch it! See how it works for yourselves! You are going to tell your friends what a fine time you had, or how high you were. You plan to repeat the moment, next time to intensify it. There is never a next time; all of this is thought. As you are walking away from the woods or wherever it is you are, you work it over in your mind, holding it to you. It is here that pleasure lives. The really interesting thing is that in this pleasure, this basking in memory, sorrow lives. For as I'm telling myself how fine I'm feeling, I've removed myself from the thrust of life. I fail to see the beauty of the hawk dropping from the sky, or smell the perfume of the woods, for I've removed myself in thought and here sorrow lives. The experience might have had an energy, a vitality of life, but it is also the case, after an experience of this sort, it's possible to judge it as unpleasant or something to be avoided. Experiences of extreme sensation or extraordinary physical danger to oneself or one's loved ones may also have a fantastic energy and a timelessness. But we don't judge them to be pleasant; we may judge them to be painful. But it is only the judgment that contains the pleasure or the pain. The experience as it is, just is. So that pleasure, or what we call pleasure, is actually a state of mind; it is not in the living relationship itself. To be a human being who is continually seeking pleasure is to be continually looking at the past, because that is where pleasure lives. Thought is what is seeking, and what it seeks is pleasure, and the pleasure itself is but thought. It is important to see this; to see how it works in oneself is what the meditative process is about.

A person who is continually seeking pleasure is a person continually in sorrow, for pleasure contains sorrow by its very nature; and to be seeking pleasure is always to be living in sorrow. How does this work? When I am reliving an experience I've created a space so that there is an experiencer who is having or has had an experience. In this separation, in the space between the experiencer and the experienced, I have removed myself from life—its newness, its challenge. Life is a movement and when there is this space between me and it, I have removed myself from the living energy. As I am walking down the trail remembering the glory of the sunrise, I am not seeing the leaves around me, smelling the freshness of the air, whatever is happening, because I have removed myself in memory. In this space what I've created is sorrow. You know the feeling of not ever being or having enough: that I am not good enough, not true enough, nor rich enough—spiritually or experientially. The truth about pleasure is you never get enough, no matter how much you get it is not enough.

Pain is not any different from pleasure. Pleasure and pain are two sides of a coin. And there is much pleasure in pain: the memory, the nostalgia, the bittersweetness, the self-pity, all of the things I squeeze from my daily living. There is pleasure here, and great sorrow.

The mind is so clever, thought is so sly. It says, "Well, all right. I see this. I see that pleasure contains sorrow and to seek anything means seeking pleasure, which is sorrow. So I'll stop seeking pleasure or try to train myself not to seek it through one discipline or another." Why do I want to do this? Don't I feel that if I can stop seeking pleasure, which is sometimes called having desires, then new and wonderful, more sublime, more, spiritual pleasures will come my way? Of course this is just another elaborately disguised seeking of pleasure. The desire to be desireless is but another desire.

Out of belief I may create hierarchies of desires and evaluate them according to my conditioning—"low" desires for material gain or power or sensuality, "high" desires for God and spirituality. Are there "high" and "low" desires, or is there not just desire that hooks onto anything? Looking at pleasure there seems to be no way out of it. If I try to get out of it, the trying itself puts me back in. So what can I do?

The question is whether or not it's possible for an ordinary human being, not a saint or a master or a guru, to see how this whole process works, and in the seeing itself to move in such a way that pleasure is no longer a problem in living. Is it possible? That's what we are going to look at. Of course, if I should tell you it's possible and you believed me, we'd just be involved again in belief. It's important to find out for yourself if it's actually possible to come into direct contact with the nature of pleasure—to see it. For to see it is to see yourself, and the seeing contains within it its own movement.

One of the great problems of the world is that the older I get and the more experiences I have tasted, the more I hunger for something greater, something new, something more intense. The more jaded I become in my pleasures the more I look for new greater ones. Spirituality, to be next to God, or to be God in oneself—these I come to view as the greatest possible pleasures. In all of this is great sorrow. In the very nature of the seeking of all of this, sorrow lives. Is it possible to be free, totally free of this? A freedom that is not a function of seeking anything else, a freedom that is different?

Pleasure and belief are interrelated. How much pleasure I get from a belief conditions me to that belief. I believe in capitalism, or communism, or Catholicism, or Hinduism, or Protestantism, and this belief makes me better than you who do not believe as I do. If I'm a Moslem and you a Christian, I think it's better to be a Moslem. If I felt it were better to be a Christian, I'd be one. Of course, I get extraordinary pleasure out of being better than you, or I can feel sorry for you, or pity you in your wrongness, or your stupidity, whatever. One can observe the whole nature of dominance in terms of beliefs. My belief makes me a little better, superior to you.

See how much energy, how much time you spend each day building structures that make you feel better than others. But the energy that is put into feeling superior negates life. Each time I convince myself I am better than you, which is a great pleasure, I have dulled myself with fragmentation, which is the root of sorrow. I pick my beliefs insofar as they will give me pleasure or allay fear, which we will examine later. Beliefs and the pleasure I get from them fragment me. They separate me from you, and as they do so they create extraordinary sorrow because of the separation. To see this, not try to make it go away, not to negate it, just to see the way it works, is a vital inroad into the nature of oneself.

I seek, and I see that I seek pleasure. I see that in the seeking of pleasure I'm continually creating sorrow. I want to stop, but the very wanting to stop is another way of seeking pleasure, so there's great conflict. To approach the question of what is one to do, we must examine the whole nature of conflict, freedom, and choice.

Question. You talk of watching pleasure but doesn't that mean you have separated yourself from it, making what you call an experiencer who is separated?
Answer. There are two ways of observing something. I can watch a river by sitting on the bank such that I'm removed from the river and watch it flow by; all I get is a picture of a river from one point, as it were, so there's removal. Or I can observe the river by being in it and flowing with it. That's the kind of observation I'm talking about, which is not a removal, which is not being in a vacuum, which is actually a living process. I can only observe the whole nature of pleasure as I'm actually involved in the living of it, which means not to try to make it go away or change it, but to watch it and see how it works, to see just what it's all about. Here the watcher and the watched are not separate. When I observe totally the nature of pleasure, which lives in thought, I observe the pleasure is me, so there is no separation, no removal from it or trying to change it. It's different—it's just a shift of awareness.

Question. Doesn't the observing of pleasure bring pleasure?
Answer. Anything may bring pleasure. If in the seeing of pleasure thought comes in and says "My, how aware I am," then there is pleasure. Here too there is a separation of seer and seen.

To glory in the memories of one's previous awareness is nothing but playing in memory.

Question. You said that pain lives in the mind. When I fall or burn myself it hurts. You can say it's in the mind all you want—it still hurts.

Answer. Certainly, the nerves feel. The feeling, as it is occurring, may be quite intense. You may not like it, wish it did not happen, and desire it to be gone. When I use the word "pain," what I'm talking about is what the mind does with the feelings. The feelings themselves are what they are. What some call pain, others may call pleasure. One actually contains the other, for in pleasure there is sorrow and in sorrow there is pleasure. The pain that intense feeling may bring twists into the pleasure of self-pity, or is utilized for one excuse or another.

Question. What I hear you saying is that pleasure and pain are the way the mind judges an experience, but I am not convinced. It seems to me that some experiences are intrinsically painful, burning yourself for example, and some are intrinsically pleasant, like sex. Or if one is hungry and eats, the cellular satisfaction that is felt is pleasure, and it's not all in my head, although I agree that thought can intensify it. Maybe there are two kinds of pleasure—mental and physiological. Why not differentiate: call one Pleasure A and the other B; or call mental pleasure ego pleasure, which I agree does bring sorrow but still leaves room for intrinsic pleasure.

Answer. If you put your hand on a hot stove, certainly there is feeling, intense feeling, which you may call pain. The calling it pain is not the feeling. At the instant the hand touches the stove, all there is is feeling of the sort that the body by its nature moves away from unless otherwise conditioned. If sufficiently intense, the experience leaves its mark in your mind as memory and in the cells themselves as burned tissue with their own feeling. If we look carefully at it when we call this feeling pain, what we are doing is evaluating it. The feeling just is what it is. In some very fundamental way, the evaluation that creates time is the pain. Pain can only live in time, in the memory of what was and the anticipation of what will be. You see, the physiological state that the fear of pain creates is a part of pain. The pain is not the feeling that is now, but the feeling coupled with the fear of its continuance.

Most of us have been conditioned to the word "pleasure" in such a fashion that it is at the central core of our lives. Should someone come and say that pleasure is not all it's made out to be, we still battle for it and are loath to remove it from the prominent part it plays. Are there mental pleasures and intrinsic pleasures? Is the question itself semantic, that is to say—merely verbal? Many people seem to consider sexuality, and by this they mean copulation and orgasm, which is only one aspect of sexuality, a great pleasure in and of itself. Eating when one is hungry, which is satisfying a biological urge or returning homeostatically to within certain boundaries is often looked at as a basic pleasure. I suppose that by "basic" or "intrinsic pleasure" one means that anytime it occurs, unless mitigated by overriding circumstances, there is good feeling. Certainly copulation or eating contains feeling, but is the feeling intrinsically good? That is to say—does one necessarily like it? Is the feeling and the liking of the feeling the same? What I'm saying is that the feeling just is what it is, having an experience instead of being the experience. When we look at the nature of death we will see how pleasure is a way of supporting personality. We are greedy: not only do we want to experience but we want to know we are having it. It is here that pleasure comes in.

There are moments in life that are marked by a quality of energy that does not live in time, wherein there is no fragmentation, no separation between the experiencer and the experience. Bliss or serenity is what this is usually called. It is not a possession; one cannot have it. After the fact, one may like or dislike it, creating a pleasure or sorrow. Bliss is not a pleasure; we only think it is, out of the memory of it.

CHAPTER 3

FREEDOM

I want to be free. At least, I think I want to be free. I have many ideas about what it is to be free. I think the way the word *freedom* is ordinarily used involves having many alternatives, many choices. The freer I am, the more choices I have. By exercising the thing called free will, or whatever you call it, I choose. The more choices I have, the freer I am; so I look for life with more and more choice in it, and I consider that to be freedom. Isn't that the way we ordinarily think about freedom? But to be truly free in the only meaningful way the word "freedom" can ever be used is to have no choice at all, which is freedom in action. Let us examine this.

If I have a choice about anything—should I go to this movie or that movie, should I do this job or that, should I marry this man or that, should I go to Hawaii or Canada for a vacation, or whatever the choice is, it doesn't matter at all. What is always there? What lives in choice? Conflict lives there, doesn't it? I don't know what to do, so there is choice. If I knew what to do there would be no choice, no conflict. In any situation of choice there is always conflict. Should I do this or that? Please look at it in yourselves and see what happens when there is choice. See how action is frozen, bound in conflict. The important thing is to see how it works in you. If there were no conflict, there would be no choice. Since there is in this world today extraordinary conflict, so there appear to be extraordinary choices. We move from one choice to the other trying to resolve our conflicts. But any movement that is done out of conflict only creates more conflict.

23

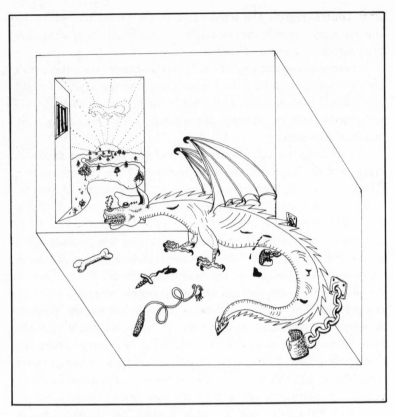

Seeing the Nature of his creation moves Memry

Look, I am a young man. I want to paint pictures. My parents want me to be a doctor. Doctors make money; artist don't. My parents will support me in medical school, but not in art school. I don't know what to do; there is conflict. The pressure is mounting because the school term starts soon. I must choose. The medical school accepts me and I go there. I have made a choice with effort and now it's over. There is an initial release of tension. Fifteen years go by and I realize that I never really liked being a doctor, but now what can I do? I made a choice out of conflict and for years I have been living with it. That is just an example of how much of life is lived in this fashion. Whenever an action is done out of conflict you can tell, for there is always a residue of thought. The residue is, of course, regret. The mind plays in the "what ifs" of bypass choices. Regret lives in the mind and is an indication that action has been forced as a result of conflict.

Where does conflict come from? Conflict comes when there isn't clarity in seeing what is. If there is a clarity in seeing what is and if I am in direct confrontation with what is, then there is no conflict. I see something clearly, directly, immediately, so that the seeing is the action of movement.

I'm walking through the forest. Suddenly there's an explosive crack, and the huge tree above me is falling. I see this—I see it is falling. To see the tree falling is to move. There is no choice, no conflict. I don't say, "Should I move, or should I not move?" Is the tree falling on me, or is it not falling on me?" If I do this, the tree is going to hit me. To see the tree falling is to move. It is not that first I see and then through a decision, a rational process I move. To see is to move—immediately. The seeing is the movement.

I'm walking down a beach and out a couple of yards is a very young child. The child is splashing around. To see the child is drowning is to move. If I say to myself, "Should I or should I not try to save the child, is he actually drowning or is he playing?" then the child could drown. You may say any number of possible things when you don't see the nature of what is. To see the child drowning is to move. The seeing is the movement. The seeing clearly of an immediate physical danger is relatively easy. The situation has a demand, an urgency about it; all of your being is alive, alert, What of psychological dangers, the subtle complexities of living? There are psychological dangers that are just as real as a tree falling. I do not move from them because I do not see them. My vision is clouded by conditioning, by fear, so that I do not see the urgency of the living situation. To see a psychological danger with a clarity and directness, to see its urgency, is to move from it. The seeing is the movement.

I, however, do not see clearly. There is enormous conflict in my life. I want to be free of it, but I see that anything I do to try to free myself of the conflict comes from the conflict itself and simply creates more conflict. I do not have clarity. What am I to do? When one sees all of this, effort stops. If I see I am not clear, that is a clarity. I see I am in conflict and anything I try to do creates more conflict. In the seeing of conflict there is clarity. When there is conflict, to ask for there not to be conflict removes me from what is, namely that I am in conflict, and puts me into ideas, beliefs of what I should be—having no conflict. That just creates more conflict. In the space between the *is* and the *ought* lives conflict. Are you following this? It sounds involved, but really it's simple. It just involves seeing it totally.

A really interesting thing about seeing clearly is that clarity is its own movement. I'm in conflict about anything: I'm a young man. Should I or should I not register for the draft? If I register for the draft they are going to come and get me and make me kill people whom I have nothing against. If I don't register for the draft they may catch me and put me in jail. I don't want to go to jail, and I don't want to kill anybody—so there is conflict.

That is just one example; there are innumerable others in living. When one begins to see the nature of what is, to see it, the seeing is its own movement psychologically. Just as to see a tree falling upon you is to move physically, so, too, to see a psychological danger is to move. And in the seeing there is no conflict, no choice, just movement. Real freedom involves the clarity of seeing what is, and it is only when clarity is there, that there is action without conflict.

Most of us seek peace, and by peace what we ordinarily mean is some state of equilibrium in which we are not affected by the trials and tribulations of the world. When we say *peace*, what we are actually asking for is removal. What real peace is—which has nothing to do with any ideas one has about peace, which is not a turning off of life—is action without conflict. To move in the world without conflict, to move freely, is to be at peace. But how do I do it? How do I manage this in a world of incredible tension, extraordinary violence, and seemingly endless sorrows? In this world of demands and fantastic desires, how does peace come?

In order for there to be movement without conflict, I must see. To see the world at all, I must see myself. How can I see the world through a dirty lens? I cannot actually see another human being in relationship unless I know the vehicle that is seeing; in short, unless I know myself. So, to see that I have conflict, neither to accept nor deny the conflict, nor to try to make it go away, but to see it, to see how it affects me totally, to see its roots and its seeds in my conditioning—to see all this is to bring a clarity into what I am. From the seeing of conflict, which is a clarity, movement comes. The movement may not be what you want or expect, but movements come when there is seeing, including seeing the fact that I'm in conflict. Just as a tree that is falling upon me is a physical danger, and to see it is to move; so, too, is conflict a great psychological danger in living. To see it as such is to move. The whole trick is in the seeing. And that, of course, is a moment to moment thing, because what I am is a living being, a flowing being.

Question. Isn't conflict at times freedom? For example, whether to go to Canada or Hawaii?
Answer. What I have been saying is that this is the way freedom is ordinarily used. I have the freedom to decide if I'm going to Canada or Hawaii, marry this lady or that, but in actual situations, if there is conflict is there freedom?

I have just been left a large sum of money; many new possibilities (choices) appear to open up. Should I take a trip? If so, where? Should I leave my job? Buy this or that? So I say that new freedom out of these choices has come my way. There doesn't appear to be any problem or conflict, yet there seem to be many choices. If I look at it closely I see that this is not a situation containing real choice, so, of course, there is no conflict. For what I am calling choice is just thought dwelling in pleasure, in the anticipation of fulfilling desires. I am not really concerned with what I am going to do. I'm just lost in the pleasure, the idea of being able to do many things. Should pressures bring about real choice, then conflict comes.

I'm not looking at the ideas we have about freedom. I'm looking at the actuality of what I am, and when there is conflict about what I ought or ought not to be doing, is there freedom? I may have the idea that, yes, I am free and that somewhere from within my internal structure I have the power to do this or that. But that's just an idea. I am talking about the living fact that I am in conflict and all of what I conceive to be freedom is just thought as it plays with itself, creating more conflict.

Question. Are you a free person?

Answer. Suppose I told you I'm free. Would you believe me? Suppose I told you I'm not free. Would you believe that? What difference does it make? What I am or am not doesn't matter at all. Whether I am or am not a living example of anything I am saying is superfluous, and you could speculate endlessly about whether I am or not, but it doesn't matter at all for you. What does matter is how you see yourself. That is the whole thing that really matters. The important thing is to see for yourself whether my words are true or not true, not what I myself am.

The question is whether or not it's possible to be a human being who does not move in fear, because if one is free, there is no fear. Fear binds freedom. Is it possible to be a human being who operates without conflict? Is it possible for there to be a clarity in seeing the world such that the very seeing is action that does not have with it the dross of regret or guilt? Is that possible for an ordinary human being? You must answer that question for yourself. What we are discussing is the fact that when there is freedom there is never decision.

Any action at all that is done through effort in order to resolve a conflict only creates more conflict. The only time there isn't more conflict created is when the action is effortless and the action is only effortless when there is no choice. When there is a seeing, there's a total involvement, a total relationship, as in those moments when the experiencer is not different from the experience. In the seeing there is clarity—and this only occurs when there is passion, and by passion I mean abandonment, self-abandonment. Only when there is real passion, a real giving away of all of this—my hopes, my desires, my life, me—can I ever be in relationship.

All living is challenge and response. To be alive is to be living in challenge and response. The challenge, by the very nature of challenge, is always new, always different. The tree falls, but it never falls exactly the same way twice. If the response is to be adequate, then it must also be new and fresh. Because most of us are responding almost completely out of habit, out of the past, the response is not adequate. When it is not adequate we remember it, we hold it in memory. You can see this. "I should have done this, I should have done that. If only I had said this. Maybe I should have gone there. I regret this or that."

Regret is a function of inadequacy of response, and the reason is that the response comes totally from conditioning. In other words, such and such has worked for me one time, and I apply this to the new situation. But the situation is new. In order for the response to be adequate, it too must be new. An inadequate response based totally on the conditioning of the past creates conflict. One is not responding to what is but rather to ideas that one has coming out of the past. These ideas separate you from the world. They fragment you—which is conflict. The inadequate response creates more memory in the form of regret and guilt so that you are even more laden; it is even more difficult to respond totally to incoming challenge. Conflict feeds on itself. The more you act out of conflict, the more conflict you create. All of this lives in thought—all of it.

Question.   Are you saying that we should never respond from the past? If you move from a falling tree it's because you know it will kill you if it hits you. That comes from the past. I don't understand what you are saying.

Answer.   Of course our experience, which is conditioning, is a factor in any movement, for this conditioning is me. I know that a falling tree will hurt me. It's not a belief, it has come from being in the world. Obviously an infant would not see it totally. Part of the total seeing of the falling tree is the understanding that falling trees are dangerous. By understanding I mean something personal, firsthanded. You being totally what you are, and the tree being what it is makes the living relationship. In the relationship you don't "know" which way to move or whether to stand still—which is also a movement. Here, in the movement itself, if you operate from past conditioning or programming, you are not responding to the tree so the response cannot be complete. The response is a movement into the unknown. I'm not saying one should or must renounce one's conditioning, which is absurd, for how can one renounce oneself? Rather, the creative movement, which is a total response to challenge, to what's happening, is a movement out of and beyond one's conditioning so something totally new occurs. This is true of physical and psychological movement. Of course, the movement itself conditions you so that when another challenge occurs total movement jumps from that, too. Living totally is a moment to moment thing, a continual thrust out of the old into the new. It is the seeing that is the thrust. When this occurs you do not hold it in thought by remembering it; you are right there to meet the next challenge. If the response is not adequate, which means that it comes totally out of past conditioning, or is bound in conflict, you hold on to it in memory with regret or guilt, so that your energy is absorbed in the past. Much of our energy is absorbed in the past and it increases as we age, making total response very difficult. Seeing all of this is a clarity that brings forth its own response, its own movement.

Question.　How will total response solve my problems?

Answer.　What we want, what we think peace is, is a life without problems, but life without problems would be a dull thing. The problem is not that there are problems, the real problem is that I do not respond to my problems completely. Real peace is not a life without problems. When the problems of living are met totally and creatively, so that one is free to move on to the next challenge, there is peace. It is only through meeting problems that growth occurs.

Question.　Should we stop wanting to change—since wanting to change causes conflict?

Answer.　I'm not saying we should or shouldn't want to change. The fact is we do want to change. Isn't that it? To say to oneself, "I shouldn't want to change because if I don't want to change, then maybe something good will happen to me" is just to be in the whole thing again. If you want to change you can observe exactly what it means to want to change, which is being in conflict. "Here is what I am. Here's what I want to be." There's a gap. I can observe this and to observe the conflict is to watch oneself. It's not changing the fact that one wants to change, but watching the fact that one does want to change, and what it does to living—that brings movement. That brings real change.

Question. Why couldn't it be true that when one is responding to a falling tree there is still choice, but the choosing is quicker, in milliseconds perhaps. At the time, choosing may not be on a conscious level. You talk about the seeing and the movement being one, but physically, that is not the way it works. It takes the time—however short—for the lightwaves to get to you, more time to reach the brain, then more time for the brain's messages to reach the muscles. Why in all of this is there not time for choice?

Answer. I think that you are asking, "Doesn't it take time, however quick, to see, and is there not more time between the seeing and the response? And, if this is so, then there is time for choice in all instances of response." Is that what you are asking?

Questioner. Yes.

Answer. Certainly the physiological models we use to explain behavior all have time as an element. In fact the nature of intellectual explanation necessarily contains time, going from here to there takes time, causes bring about effects only in time, and so forth. Yet even in physical science the nature of time is not such a clear-cut thing. From an inward, an internal point of view, does seeing ever occur in time? We have an idea that there is something external out there that we perceive and internalize, and the process occurs in time. Let us look at the nature of the internal and the external. Most of us consider the skin and everything inside of it as internal and everything outside of it as external. The internal is "me," and external "not me." There is a bird singing in a tree. Where is the sound of the bird? Is it in the vocal chords of the bird? In the air waves as they touch my ear? In the tympanic membrane? Along the auditory nerves or in the brain itself? Where is the sound of the bird—out there or in me? Internal or external? Actually, the sound is neither in the bird nor in me, but rather in the total relationship. When there is total relationship, at that instant, the division between the internal and external is not there. It is thought that creates the division which creates the "me" and the "not me." Time lives in the division between "me" and "not me."

When there is sound it does not take time to hear the sound. There is just sound. When one sees anything, there is no time. Here, by "seeing," I do not mean just sensory input, although it certainly includes that. I am talking about a total relationship.

Does the response that comes with relationship take time? Only when thought looks back at it does time enter. The seeing is the response; they are not separate. Only thought in trying to understand, which means to recognize, separates perception from action. Newness can never be recognized. Only the old, the known, is recognizable. The seeing of challenge, which by its nature is new, and the response to it are not divided. They are one. Thought, which after the fact wants to explain the response, creates time by putting the explanation in causal terms. That is, it makes the challenge the cause, and the response the effect. Thought which is mechanical can explain only in mechanistic terms. In fact, to be in thought is necessarily to be in time. That is something we will look at later. Seeing totally, which never occurs in time, has its own movement, which is choiceless.

CHAPTER 4

FEAR

I am afraid of many things: of being hurt, of not living fully, of not realizing myself to my fullest potential, of not being spiritually aware. I am afraid of death, of loneliness, of losing the securities I have. I am afraid that the pleasures I had yesterday will no longer be tomorrow. I'm afraid my loved ones won't love me; I am even more afraid that I won't love them. There is great fear in living. Ordinarily what we do with fear is invent systems, beliefs, to try to make it go away. But fear is all-pervading. It is there from minute to minute. I can try to forget about it; I can pretend it doesn't exist, but it is there. It influences so much of my movement.

I am walking down the street with my friend and a stranger comes up to me and insults me. Instead of responding to him directly, I hold back because my friend might think I'm boorish and not like me. So there are social fears of not being liked or accepted. I want something from you: your attention, your affection, your concern. I want some special privilege. So, when you come to me, instead of relating to you immediately, I hold back out of my desires, out of my wants.

Fear and ambition are always linked. If there were no ambition, no desire, there would be no fear. If you didn't want anything, would there be anything to be afraid of? There is only fear when you want something—something you don't have, or have and don't want to lose. Isn't that where fear lives? I have a love today; I'm in love; I want to make sure this love lives with me tomorrow, so I begin doing things to secure it, and fear comes. I want to

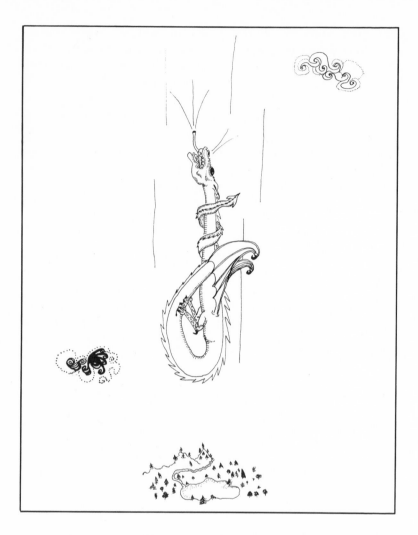

Memry strangles his Self

live forever because I'm afraid of death, and fear comes. I want you to like me, so I operate in certain ways out of fear. I'm not saying you should or shouldn't do this. We are just looking at the nature of fear. When there is fear there is always ambition. When there is ambition, fear is there. As soon as you want something, a part of that want is the fear you won't get it. To see fear in the day-to-day process of living, and to see that where there's ambition there's fear, is to get into the nature of thought. It is thought that wants. It is thought that is very ambitious. My family, my country, my life, all of these have to do with what I want.

I tend to treat fear as an external thing—as if there is something outside of me that has come in and taken me over. But the reality of it is that when there is fear, I am fear. It's not that I'm having fear—fear is me. For most of us in day-to-day living, there is fear. Fear that everything we have lived for is going to fall down and break apart. It is only if we can actually begin to live with fear, which is not to try to make it go away, but live with it from moment to moment, that fear can be a teacher, psychologically.

Fear can teach me about myself. If I want something from you, I can observe what the wanting, the ambition does in our relationship. The sound of my voice and the tensions in my body reflect the ambition even if it is simply wanting you to like me. To see the way it works is to see how fear is a part of what I ordinarily consider relationship to be. To see how fear is always linked with ambition, and to see how the ambition itself generates fear, so that actually ambition and fear are not different—this seeing brings forth movement, the seeing *is* the movement. Fear is as great a psychological danger to living as a tree falling is a physical danger. To see it is to move.

From a very early age I have been conditioned to ambition, by society and by parents. Society wants us to produce; our parents want to be proud of us so they can take pleasure in identification. All of this is very competitive, for I only gauge success in competitive terms. I only know if I'm good or successful if I'm better than you. Schools condition us this way, too, with A's and B's. What it is to be a *good* human being comes from beliefs conditioned into me, so that ambitions aim toward nothing more than conditioned beliefs. We saw earlier how beliefs contain violence within them. Ambition, fear, belief, violence, these are just aspects of living that most of us act out daily.

Fear freezes action, for when there is fear there is also conflict. In a physically dangerous situation, if one thinks of the possible outcomes, one is frozen and here is where fear lives. I don't want to die or lose an arm or leg, so here is ambition, a concern of what will be, which removes the energy from what is, and while it occurs I am immobile, in conflict. What is, is danger. What I want to be is safely out of it, and here there is fear. The same is true regarding our psychological problems. In psychological conflict, am I not afraid that I will make a wrong choice, or that to go one way is to miss out on more profound experiences? I am so afraid of missing out! All of this binds me. Fear isn't pleasant, so I want to make it go away. In the very act of trying to make fear go away, which is just another ambition, I create more of it. As I get older and older I become more fearful. I begin to look back and see my life slipping away as the pleasures that once engrossed me become stale, and I look for something deeper. I'm afraid that I'm never going to be fulfilled, that my life is going to slip past and nothing is going to happen.

Is it possible for a human being to be free of fear? When there is fear, when I'm afraid, there cannot be any learning. Fear and learning never live side by side. If I'm afraid to look, afraid that what I see I won't like or will not be acceptable to me or won't fit into my system of beliefs, then I have removed myself from learning.

Is it possible to live and not be enmeshed continually in fear? In order to answer that question for yourself, you must get to know fear. Get to know it and see how it works. See where its seeds live. See how the seeds live in the past and are always projecting into the future, because fear only lives with concern for the future. Fear is very egocentric, which is not to say it's good or bad, just that fear is always involved with *my* pleasures, *my* experiences. Am I going to get enough? Are the pleasures that I have going to continue? Fear is a great teacher—psychologically. To watch fear, to attend to it, to try neither to make it go away nor to bring it about, to just watch it work, is to learn about yourself. Fear is the opener of doors. For to be the fear, which is not to be running away from it, but to be living it, so that the fear is me, is a change in awareness, a turn of mind.

I am walking down the street. It is late at night and a man comes and asks me for a light. I am fearful of him. I can listen to the sound of my voice and I can hear the way I respond. I am trying to make him go away. What does he want from me? I can feel the adrenalin flowing. I can feel the tightening of my viscera. I can feel the manifestation of the thought, "This man may want to hurt or kill me." The fear expresses itself in the sound of my voice, in movements of my body. There is fear in so much of living, in so much of what we call relationship, not only with the stranger but with my husband or wife, lover or child. I am afraid you won't like me, or please me, or clean my house when the boss comes to dinner. Out of these needs or ambitions, comes fear. To be aware of it is to be learning from it. What do I want? What am I interested in, in this fearful situation? I don't want to be hurt. I don't want to lose what I have—a comfortable life, a wife who is a servant, my standing in the community, my life—all of which breeds fear.

Please understand, I am not suggesting that we try to throw away ambition in order to do away with fear. I am not saying that ambition is good or bad or that it should or should not be. Nor am I saying that I should want to be hurt, or not want to be hurt. The turn to awareness that I'm talking about is a way of seeing the totality of what is—by living it.

All of the organized religions play with fear and play with belief. If you believe what I tell you and do what I tell you, then I will allay the basic fears you have about death, about the meaningfulness of living. I will give you answers you want to hear. All of this, whether it be the promise of heaven, the promise of a better next life, or whatever organized religions promise, it's all playing with fear. I believe them out of fear, because I want something—security. Fundamentally, all these fears are wrapped around one basic thing—fear of the unknown. I am very afraid of the unknown.

Fear also plays with pleasure. One can observe as one moves from one pleasure to another that there is always the fear of not holding on to it, of not getting more of it, of it not being enough. So I continue out of fear, trying to recapture the old experiences, which is security. All of this lives in thought. Fear lives in thought. Fear actually is thought as it plays in the past, as it projects into the future, as it plays in time. For to be in time, to be living in time as we do, is to be living in fear, as we do. One cannot put down fear, just as one cannot put down ambition or desire. It's there. I may try to make fear go away because I'm afraid that I'll miss something if fear stays with me. I'll miss some great experience or some way of being. Fear operates in the mind always. If it is there, to try to put it away is just to increase it, so here again is another bind of mind. The more I try to make fear go away, the more I'm continually creating it. So once again, as I look at this, I see that anything I try to do only re-creates the very thing I'm trying to escape, which is fear. So what am I to do?

First, get to understand fear, to see it. But here there is another trick of mind. I say, "Yes. I'm going to try and understand it." And I try to look at it, but I'm always looking at it with an eye to trying to make it go away. If I see it properly, then perhaps it will go away. That isn't looking at it at all. That's just being involved again in an idea, in a hope, ambition.

The intimate direct relationship of being one's fear so that one sees it clearly, sees the way it works, sees its psychological danger and how it kills every moment by putting me in the past and projecting me into the future, that seeing brings movement. To see the sorrow in fear as it removes me from direct living enables a movement to come about. It is no different than seeing totally a falling tree; the seeing is the movement. So to see fear totally, as the psychological danger that it is, is to move. But if I look in order to move, I'm not looking. I'm just ambitious.

All of what we have been talking about—beliefs, pleasure, ambition, freedom, and fear—are linked together in some very fundamental way. To see the way they operate, to observe them, is to see the nature of thought.

Real learning, real inquiry, real freedom, does not live when there is fear. If I am afraid that to see myself I'll not like what I see, then I won't look. If I'm afraid that inquiry may remove me from the pleasures I'm familiar with, then growth stops. To see the way fear works, to see it as a psychological danger to living, to see it as a handmaiden to sorrow, to see it, not to try to make it go away, but just to see it, which means to live with it directly, in my movement, in the sound of my voice, from moment to moment—it is only then that one can be free of fear. It does not come by asking to be free of it, or by having any ideas about what freedom from it means, but only by living with it can freedom come, a freedom that is different from anything that one seeks.

Question. Are most of your thoughts about fear negative?

Answer. I never said fear was bad. I am simply observing the way fear works, which is very different than having thoughts about it. Much teaching is done in terms of fear. If a toddler is in the road he may get run over. I don't want that to happen so I teach my child to be afraid of the road. In terms of teaching, of how to live in the world, the teaching of fear itself is not a survival mechanism, actually. Out of fear, I forbid my child to do many things, so that he never learns how to survive as an organism. Learning is only response to challenge. If out of fear I remove the challenges from children or anyone, then the organism doesn't grow and flourish. Mostly I'm not afraid for my child at all. I'm afraid for myself. I'm afraid my child will get hurt or die and leave me and I won't like that. Again what we're dealing with is linked with ambition. I want my child to be a certain way, which means I must promulgate fear. Again it is me, for to do this is not for the child, but for me. That isn't to say one should leave an infant on the road, which of course is absurd. The nature of being very young makes some protection necessary— obviously. To know what challenges are appropriate for a given child is the challenge of being a parent or a teacher. There is no formula. Formulas are worshipped by those who, out of fear, sidestep the continual newness of challenge. When a response is not total, it is fear that removes one from real responsibility. What responsibility actually is, is response-ability, the ability to respond. That isn't to say one doesn't learn from one's experience, but rather that real learning only occurs when fear is absent.

Question. You seem to say that fear does not help me survive, yet it is the memory of having hurt myself and the desire not to do so again that keeps me alive. It seems to me, therefore, that fear which is based on memory is quite essential to living.

Answer. Is fear essential to living? It is true that fear is the fuel most of us run on. There is the fear that if there were no fear in my life that I would hurt or kill myself. There is the fear that if there were no ambition to drive me I would vegetate and life would pass me by. I think that I move from a falling tree only because I don't want to get hit. I'm afraid of getting hit and that moves me. Should there be no fear, what then will move me? Let's examine this closely to see if fear is actually necessary.

First, it's important to see that it's literally not possible to be afraid of anything that is happening. If I point a gun at you, you are not afraid that I'm pointing a gun at you. You're afraid I'm going to shoot you. If I have shot you, you're not afraid of being shot; you're already shot. You're afraid that I will shoot you again or that you will bleed to death or be scarred or whatever. So fear is never a response to what is, but rather what will be out of memories of what was. So when there is fear, my energy is removed from what is. If "what is" is danger, fear removes my response-ability to the danger and there is much greater likelihood of succumbing to the danger.

Now one may say that even if all this is true, does not fear keep me out of dangerous situations? Fear may keep me out of situations that are known dangers and also keep me away from exploring the unknown. I broke my leg in an automobile accident. As a result I may stay out of automobiles totally; I may stay away from all conveyances. This is so. The question is not whether fear can keep me out of danger, but rather is fear necessary for living? Certainly I can to some extent keep danger out by enclosing myself and narrowing my life. Yet living is dangerous. The new always presents itself, and if I have not continually built strength by responding to challenge—which is what learning and growth are about—then when danger comes, whether physical or psychological, fear binds me. If through fear I remove myself from challenge and attempt to make my life secure, then I become dull and habit-bound, which is perhaps one of the greatest psychological dangers.

Now I think the real question is whether or not it's possible to be free of fear, which means to be free of one's conditioning. To be free of one's conditioning is not to negate or attempt to destroy one's conditioning. Can conditioning destroy itself? We bring to every instant the sum total of our conditioning, not only our experiences, but genetic conditioning as well. Being free of one's conditioning is not destroying this. To see a falling tree is based upon conditioning, and the movement of my body, that is the response, is based upon conditioning. Obviously a two-month-old infant would not be response-able to the falling tree. So that to be free of one's conditioning is not a negation or destruction of the conditioning, but rather a movement out of it in the living moment of response. In the moment of freedom that is timeless, one springs out of everything that one is. Here is where growth comes from—the creative response to challenge. Of course this jump itself becomes conditioning when memory wraps around it. Freedom then is a moment to moment thing. Fear destroys freedom. See in yourself if fear is actually beneficial in living.

While we have been looking at fear or belief or pleasure, we have also been looking at the nature of thought, the nature of meditation, because all of what we have been examining lives in thought. To see fear totally, one sees in it beliefs, pleasures, conflicts. To see conflict totally is to see fear. To see any one of them clearly, totally, is to see them all; it is seeing myself. All of this lives in me and though I continue to fragment myself with thought, I am actually not fragments but a whole thing, a living thing. To see any one of the so-called fragments of thought clearly is to see it all.

We looked at belief and we saw how belief and violence are not actually different from each other, and how to be in the state of belief is to be violent. There is no difference. We looked at pleasure and we saw how to be continually seeking pleasure (and to be seeking anything at all is to be seeking pleasure) is always to be seeking the known, the past joys, something that we had and later judged to be worthwhile. To be seeking pleasure is always to be creating sorrow, continually creating the gap between the "is" and the "ought," the seer and the seen, so that there is separation, and, of course, in this separation lives sorrow and loneliness, which is quite different from being alone.

We looked at conflict, freedom, and choice and we saw how true freedom, if it has any meaning at all, is to have no choice. I am talking about internal choice, about the pressure of deciding. If you see the nature of what is, the seeing is its own movement. The seeing contains within it its own demand for action. The seeing is the action, actually. What we are doing here is looking. It is relatively easy to see the physical dangers of living, but the psychological dangers, the inner dangers are not so easy to see because part of being in psychological danger is the inability to look at it. The very seeing of any of these dangers, such as conflict or fear, is a movement, which by its very nature cannot be preprogrammed. If you see a tree falling, you move. You don't know beforehand whether you will move to the left or the right or up or down or perhaps even stand still, which itself is a movement. It all depends upon the nature of the danger, which is always different. So it is with psychological dangers: they are always different; you never know which way you are going to move before the movement occurs. But out of our desire for security, out of our wanting to know, we want it programmed. I want to know whether I am going to do this or that, because the fundamental fact of it is that we are also afraid of ourselves, of what we will do. Who knows what I'll do? So fear tends to compound itself.

We looked at fear, and we saw how ambition and fear always live with each other. If there is no wanting, there is no fear, but the reality of it is that there is ambition. We want this and that, the security, the knowledge that past experiences will be repeatable— there are all kinds of things we want. And if we see how fear and ambition are always linked, we see how wanting them to go away is just playing the same game again, because, as we said, the desire to be desireless is just another desire.

We think in terms of high and low desires. The desire for sensuality or for power over other human beings—we look upon those as not worthy. Whereas the desire for spirituality or peace or bliss we look upon as something worthy of a human being. Are there really high and low desires, good and bad desires, or is there just desire, which plays in all things? Desire is thought, which removes you from what is. As soon as I want something to be other than exactly what it is, then I have removed myself and created the gap between the "is" and the "ought." Here is something that is. I don't want it to be this way; I want it to be some other way. Here is where value, liking or disliking, which is again a product of thought, comes in. Likes and dislikes sap your energy.

We saw how, in order to utilize fear as the great teacher it is, one must actually be the fear, live with it as a moment to moment thing, see how it crops up, how it destroys real relationship. For when I either want or don't want something from you, the wanting of it generates fear, which removes me from you. When I walk down the street and I see the cripple or the beggar or the poor person or the ugly, it doesn't please. I turn my eyes away; I would rather not see him. I turn him off. In doing so I have to turn off my environment because I'm afraid that if it's a beggar he may want something from me; or if it's a poor person, I might feel some obligation because of an idea or belief to take care of him. One can observe this for oneself in daily living: how your relationships (which of course, is living) contain fear, and how fear removes you from the verve of living, from the newness of life. To see it, which isn't to try to change it, is a shift of awareness that has its own movement.

Question. Listening to you makes me feel helpless and hopeless. When listening to you it seems to make sense, but it doesn't stay with me. It's frustrating.

Answer. One of the problems of listening to me is that we want to understand what is being said. What we usually mean by understanding is for thought to wrap around the words and turn them into a consistent or comfortable structure. Then I can say, "I have it. I understand. Now it's my possession," and I can regurgitate the "ideas" on command. The difficulty is that I'm not presenting ideas. I'm looking at what is. Thought can never possess what is, never wrap around it and own it. To truly understand these words one must understand oneself. To understand oneself is always a movement, a moment to moment thing. As soon as you say "I know myself," you are talking about the past, what you were, which now lives only in memory. To try to hold on to the words is not to listen. The words don't matter—how you see for yourself does.

Feeling hopeless and helpless is interesting. What is hope? Is not hope actually ambition, which contains pleasure? When one feels helpless that means one cannot do anything to make one's hopes come true, which is "frustrating." Frustration is conflict and its attendant fears.

Question.   Much of what you say doesn't seem to follow necessarily. There seems to be a sense in it, but it seems to me that the way you look at things is one possible way out of many. In listening to you I get a feeling of surety, which might be called rigid or dogmatic. When the mind is trying to see into the nature of its own workings, how it sees is limited by its own perspective. What you are saying could easily be just one way of looking at things. How do you know that what you are saying isn't just that?
Answer.   You talk as if with mind there are an infinite possible number of ways of looking at things and then ask, "How does one know that the way one is looking at things is more correct than any other." Is that not the question?

Questioner. Basically.
Answer.   To look at things as if there were an infinite number of ways to look at things is actually just one way of looking at things. There is another way—and that is to just look at them. If you will do this in yourself then perhaps the endless questions of intellectual justifications will cease. To need intellectual justifications of living is in itself just one way of looking at things. You see, only when the looking from any perspective ends, may one see. The question then is: Is it possible for a mind to look not only out of the cage of its conditioning, but to really look with no perspective at all? Is it possible for a mind to be free? Freedom only occurs when a mind dies to itself and in that death is free of fear. Let's look at death.

CHAPTER 5

DEATH

I am afraid to die so I look for systems of thought, for beliefs that will support me and will turn off the things I am afraid of, the things I don't want to look at in the world and in myself. I create heavens and hells—structures that will give me next lifetimes, or whatever it is I want—and I do it out of fear. The clever, the unscrupulous, power-motivated people are quite aware that the way to control me is with fear. So, because I'm afraid, I give up inquiry and take up belief. I become a very stale, stiff, habitual, and manageable human being. All of the religions, organizations, structures, which operate out of fear, offer promises of hope in exchange for my good behavior or my obedience. The promises they give are all contingent upon my being a certain way. The doors of heaven will open up to me only if I'm good and do what I'm told.

Beliefs separate me from you and from aspects of myself into Christian, Jew, Hindu, Moslem, American, Mexican, Communist, Capitalist—any of the "isms." When I become any of these "isms," I separate myself from you; it makes me better than you. It gives me pleasure, but separation is violent, whether it's external or internal. The world's external violence exists only because I'm violent, because I create the world in my own image. The more I try to change the world with effort (force), which is violence, the more violence I create. If I try to force the world into my ideas of nonviolence, it's just more violence.

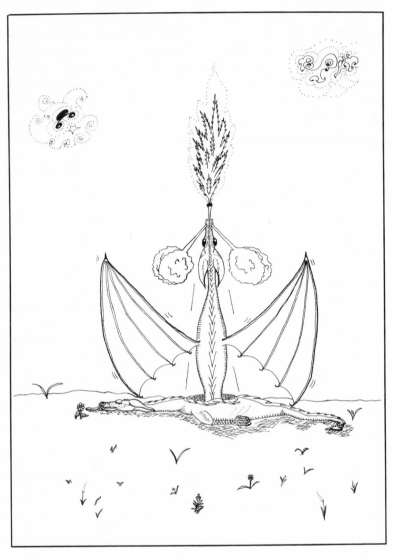

Memry's husk busts

What does all this have to do with death? Why should one concern himself with death? If one does not look at death directly, if one does not come face to face with it, then we live always in its shadow, and the shadow is fear.

What does it mean to say I'm afraid to die? Am I talking about physical death? Physical death is an abstraction; it's not anything I can know about. I see animals dying. Every now and then I see a human die, although in our society it's very well hidden from us, and from this I project the fact that I, too, am going to die and physically disintegrate. But all of this is abstract, quite removed and remote. Yet I'm afraid of death. Exactly what am I afraid of?

Isn't it true that what I'm really afraid of is losing myself? I'm fearful of losing that which I'm familiar with—myself, my personality, what we call ego, that which is me—that which makes me distinct from other human beings. So when I say I'm afraid to die, is it not the personality (not the so-called physical self, but the personality) that I'm afraid of losing—the me? All of the religions that promise eternal life—what do they promise? They promise the eternal life of the soul or the spirit. And what they mean, of course, is that what will continue is you, the personality.

Have you ever wondered why people believe in and seem to get security from a religion that vaguely promises heaven to a few and seems to guarantee hell to most of its followers? The answer is quite simple. Hell, too, guarantees the continuation of personality, which is preferable to total annihilation. Even hell is better than not being at all.

If I look at death and the fear of death very carefully, I see that what I'm afraid of is the fact that I (personality) am going to go away. That's what fear of dying is, that I'm not going to be anymore. Me, the person, the separate thing, the unique entity that makes me different from you, is going to die. What is this "me"? Where does personality live? Have you ever asked yourself who you are? Who are you? What is this familiar entity that you are always nurturing? Where does it live?

The answer isn't very complicated—it lives in memory. What we are is memory. You remember all of the pleasures, pains, sorrows, joys, all of the experiences of living—all of the things you internalized out of the past. That is what you are, isn't it? You say you know yourself, but what is it that you know? You know only what you have done, what you were. To call all of that "you" (or what you are) makes you feel very safe and secure. It's so comfortable. I say, "I know what I am and what I am capable of doing." For if I don't think I know what I am and what I'm capable of, then a great fear of insecurity would come in. Why, I might destroy everything I hold dear, follow this fantasy or that—ruin myself. Out of fear of the unknown (newness), I continually perpetuate the known; the known, of course, is my personality. The perpetuation of the known is habit, which brings dullness.

In situations of extraordinary conflict, where we don't know what we are going to do, we have all kinds of ideas about what we could or ought to do, or what a good or brave or worthy human being would do. Then we're afraid that perhaps we'll be different from the image we have of ourselves. I'm afraid that if physical courage is demanded of me, I will turn and run. Out of fear or pleasure, we continually re-create the part of ourselves we feel safe about or the self that pleases us. The "I" or personality or ego, lives in thought. You can look at a child and see a relatively unformed personality. Then the infant grows, gathering experience, and personality begins to emerge. As we get older and older, we become more set in our personality: "I know myself, I have seen myself, I have seen the world, and I know;" and, of course, because you have said that, you are talking about something old.

It is the personality that we are forever interested in re-creating, but the personality is always something that is out of the past. And, of course, the people that we live with, our loved ones, our friends—all our relationships and the whole structure of society—program us to continue in this form. My children want the security that I am going to be tomorrow just what I am today. My husband wants the security that ten years from now I am going to love him as much as I love him now, or loved him five years ago. My government wants to be sure I'm going to be obedient and do everything it says. There are all kinds of pressures, external and internal, to freeze our personalities, making us a predictable, safe, tame beast, quite respectable.

In the moments when there isn't any gap or space between the seer and the seen, is there a personality living at that time, or is there not simply a living relationship, which is always something new, fresh, and vital?

One of the really popular phrases that has been bantered about in the last few years, which many people are striving for, is something called "ego loss." Some of the old eastern systems aiming toward ego loss speak of the individual merging with God, or total being. Ego loss has to do with dying, with the death of the ego or personality. In seeking ego loss one presumably seeks to kill the very thing one cherishes most—namely oneself. Through effort and striving can one shut down the very thing that is striving? Can one kill ambition, which lives in the personality, by having the ambition to eradicate ambition? In searching for a state of ego loss, what we really want is for the ego (ourselves) to be grander, more profound, more spiritual, which feeds the very thing (ego or personality) that presumably is to be done away with. To see that is a door to understanding death.

We tend to think that life and death are separate and different. We put them at opposite ends of a spectrum: "Here is life; when life is absent here is death." Then we build ethics or moralities and say things like, "I am a worshiper of *life*." One can, out of structure, worship death just as easily, as some religions do. The greatest promise of some systems is not to return again (to reincarnate), but to leave the wheel of life eternally.

Life and death, however, are not different or separate. They are just different ways of looking at a total movement. Every moment as I move through the world I am dying. My cells are changing—the whole process of living is dying. In order for me to live I must kill living things to eat. It is not that there is life or death, or that life comes out of death—it's that life *is* death. There is no difference. To live is to die. The very thing that I fear—losing my personality—is necessary if I'm to be in contact with the new, if I'm actually to be in contact with the living moment. How can I be in relationship with you if all I see when I see you are all of the memories we have had together. In order for me to see you as a new thing, a fresh thing, a living thing, I must die to all of the past—to all of the memories, all of the flatteries, all of the insults, all of the relationships that we have had together; in short, I must die to my personality. That actually is what ego loss is all about. But if I try to get this relationship, if I seek it, all I can seek is memory.

The living-dying process is like fire. Fire has an energy, a burning quality, but along with it there is a residue of ash. It is not that the fire causes or creates ash but rather that they are two sides of the same process. What most of us do is give enormous import to the ashes of living. The ash of life is memory. To play with ashes is to put out the fire.

I once had an experience. I remember that it was something extraordinary. There was an extraordinary delight, extraordinary life, verve, and I want to have this more often. It is not the "extraordinary moment" itself that I'm trying to recapture, for that is gone. It is the memory of the moment that has become part of me (my personality) which I'm seeking. The memory is not the thing. And, of course, to seek after it as a goal or reward is to seek after something old. When one can die to oneself, to one's personality, actually let go of the pleasures, pains, flatteries, insults, all of it—then one is in immediate contact with living, because living and dying are not different.

It has been said that ordinary day-to-day life without memory is impossible. Obviously, I must remember my name and countless things about the world I live in; I must utilize the accumulation of my experience, for that's what makes me an adult able to live in the world.

There is a place where memory as a pragmatic, practical tool has its uses, and this person is not saying that these uses are inappropriate. But there are modes of being wherein memory is not appropriate. Where memory is or is not appropriate is a function of living awareness, and that's a moment to moment thing. What meditation concerns itself with is the death of thought, which is the death of memory—actually dying, dying continually, so that one is continually reborn. For it is only then that one is in immediate contact with the living.

We are looking at the nature of thought here: thought that plays in fear, that is continually re-creating personality, ourselves. We live in our thoughts. I'm not asking you to make your thoughts go away

Actually you cannot, for thought cannot conquer itself. The important thing is to observe thought and see how it works. Only from the intimate seeing of the way we work is real change and growth possible. Otherwise we're caught in the old—always.

When there is dying, inwardly, there is passion, which literally means abandonment. To be passionate is to be abandoned, and when you abandon you let go of everything (yourself); only then does passion live. Creativity, which is responding to the challenges of the moment, responding totally in an unfettered way, creativity only occurs when there is passion, when there is caring, which is also abandonment, which is death—death of the old, death of the self.

A very interesting thing is that when we seek many of these so-called spiritual states, the seeking is an attempt to increase the very personality that must die in order for "spiritual states" to occur. That is part of the paradox of it. The more I hunger for the eternal, the more I negate it. The question is: "If everything I do in terms of effort and seeking turns on itself, what do I do?" I want to live fully, deeply, richly, yet continual seeking is negation. I'm afraid of death, yet I seek the kind of death that gives rebirth, so there's conflict. What do I do?

If you were living on a mountain top and all around you was an abyss and anywhere you moved you would fall, what would you do. First, you would stop moving and get to know the little plot you're sitting on. You would get to know it rather intimately. So it is with the nature of thought. Thought is an endless abyss that we are continually living with and cannot escape. Who is trying to escape from it? Is it not thought itself saying, "I must escape from thought?" Here is conflict. So what can I do?

As we've seen, any action that involves effort or force, only creates more conflict. So I stop and observe the nature of conflict. That's what we're doing: We're observing the whole nature of thought, because it is only when one can observe it that a quietness can possibly come. A quietness that is not mechanical, that is not a function of an asking for quietness—because who is asking? Is not the asker thought itself? Peace only comes when this whole thing quiets, including the asking for quietness. I say that I am searching for peace, for something eternal, unblemished by time. To see that what I am actually searching for are merely ideas that come from my thoughts; to see that I cannot stop searching out of effort, for that is simply searching all over again; to see it without trying to change it (for as soon as I attempt to change it, I am no longer looking)—to see this is to see what is. If I'm in conflict, to see that is to see. From this seeing, which is its own quietness, a movement without conflict may come—that is peace. It is a peace that is not a removal or withdrawal from the world. It is a peace that is an energy, a tremendous livingness, a peace that is action without conflict. It is only when I see clearly the nature of conflict that peace may come. Death and my fear of death are interesting inroads into a way of seeing that opens doors into the nature of personality, into the *me-ness*, which lives only in memory.

Question. Is not the fear of death sometimes the fear of the possible physical pain of dying?

Answer. One can hook all kinds of fear on it. But the fear of pain in dying isn't the fear of dying—it's the fear of pain. You have that same fear about hurting yourself in any fashion, don't you? Fear hooks onto anything. Because I don't want pain, because I don't like it, I become afraid. I don't want to be hurt—an ambition that brings fear. I'm not saying one should want to be hurt or not want to be hurt, nor am I examining whether it is "natural" not to want to be hurt and "unnatural" to be any other way. What, hopefully, we are doing here is observing how the whole thing works, observing it not from the outside, but totally, for I *am* my observations.

Question. Is fear of death inherent in all men?

Answer. Is fear of the destruction of oneself, not one's physical self, but one's psychological self or personality, inherent in all human beings? For me to answer that is to formulate a structure. I can only tell you what I see when I look at myself and the people around me, and the people I deal with and live with. Whether it's the case that every human being in the last 5,000 years has come to grips with it, is something I wouldn't speculate about, and it fundamentally doesn't matter. It doesn't matter if any other human being comes to grips with it or not. The only thing that does matter is you. Not what others are doing, but what you are doing. The question is, is it possible for one to actually come to terms with this in a creative way? We are going to talk about this more when we examine the nature of evolution.

Question.   You said our fear of dying involved psychological death. That may be, I'm not sure. What of physical death—the actual destruction of the body? You may say it's an abstraction, but I know it really happens. What about it?

Answer.   I did not say physical death was an abstraction. I said that fear of it was. The actuality of physical death is one of the great adventures. If one dies, psychologically, which is not a symbolic death, but a real dying, then death, which is an energy transformation, a rebirth, reveals itself. Living awareness is dying awareness.

Question.   To talk about death as transformation does not seem to differ much from the ideas of karma and reincarnation that Eastern mysticism talks of. What about that?

Answer.   In the East it is said that a person's action generates karma, or consequences, and karma determines the form of my next incarnation, or lifetime. The life I lead now is said to be a result of karma of past lifetimes. The whole structure is used to manipulate and control people. The rich or upper class tells the poor or lower class that they are miserable because they are working out past bad deeds. They are told that if they accept their misery and do as they are told, the next time around they too may be rich or powerful or saintly. Religions also derive their power and wealth from this.

I don't step on the cockroach, not because I care about the roach, but because I'm afraid that if I do I will get "bad karma." Maybe even come back in the next lifetime as a cockroach. Actually, I don't give a damn about the bug. Then too, the concept of karma is used to justify behavior. I am what I am and do what I do because it's my karma to be that way. Karma is often used as something external to justify the internal.

For me, the interesting questions about karma and reincarnation are not involved with whether they are true or false, but rather why karma or reincarnation interests me at all. There are poisons of the mind that are just as real as poisons of the body. Mind poisons are deadly not because they are totally false; if they were totally false they would be easily shucked off. They are poisonous to awareness because their very nature brings forth ambition, which removes one from life. See if you can approach your ideas about reincarnation without fear or ambition. I think most of us are interested in the continuation of personality, of ourselves. To really die inwardly, psychologically, one sees how death is transformation, for in such death, personality or the so-called ego changes and there is newness and innocence. In that transformation is adventure. The adventure of what the transformation of physical death will bring will display itself when it occurs. Why concern yourself with it? Actually, it's not possible to be concerned with that final movement, but only with ideas about it that are bred in fear and ambition. In fact, the ideas are the fear and ambition, which poison the mind.

Question. Your thoughts on mind poisons interest and confuse me. You intimate that they are poisons because they are true. How can truth be a poison?

Answer. I did not say that poisons of the mind are true. I said they are not totally false, which makes them dangerous. Most people in their many different ways are "control freaks," which is one of the ways the mind is conditioned from a very early age. We are taught to control ourselves and are rewarded for it. Then we learn to manipulate the world, and if our manipulations are successful we feel special, superior, important. So many of us are always looking for ways to feel better than others. How do I know I am any good; I know only if I'm better than you. It's all so comparative, so competitive.

We build structures of mind that we use to convince ourselves of our uniqueness. Structures are also devised that attempt to explain and therefore control our destinies; we turn to the structure for answers out of our conflict and confusion. Examples are Tarot, I Ching, Astrology. These structures have been fed energy for centuries and have been sufficiently refined so as to tap into some of the relational processes of the universe. To internalize any of these structures and view the universe out of them is to preprogram your behavior in terms of the structure. So the structure becomes a self-fulfilling prophecy.

A man I know went to a fortune teller and was told that money would come to him unexpectedly on two dates. He was also told the year of his death. Money did come to him as foretold. Now, where do you think his mind is? Can he forget the predicted year of his death? Cannot the fact of the date being placed in the mind program the body via fear to aim at that time for its demise?

People who play in these structures say that they are maps of consciousness which can teach you about yourself. A map only charts the old, the known. By looking at yourself through a structure, you are conditioning yourself to fit in it. To be free is not to fit into a structure or to utilize a structure to alleviate conflict. Freedom moves beyond any structure, beyond any conditioning.

These structures are approached out of and are fed by fear and ambition. The nature of the conditionings imposed by these systems can poison the mind and can also prevent it from seeing beyond them. An aware animal keeps away from quicksand, not because it's false but because it's deadly.

CHAPTER 6

TIME

Most of us spend a great portion of our lives fighting with time. Either there isn't enough of it and we race around trying to accomplish self or other imposed goals, or there's too much of it so that time hangs heavy on our hands and we get bored. As we grow older times seems to race by faster and faster.

For most of us. time consists of past, present, and future, and there seems to be an uncertain movement from one to the other. The movement of time from past to present to future seems elusive at best. Here we are discussing psychological time—the inward feeling of the movement of time. But where is the past? Where does the past live in you? If I were to ask you to search for the past and find where it lives in you, where would you look? Please, the important thing in these talks is to look at yourself; to see how you work. To wait passively for this person to give you answers is not inquiry. The past lives in memory, doesn't it? And what about the future? Where does it live? It lives in thought, too. The future is the past as it projects the experiences I have had into the experiences I want to have or don't want to have, which, again, is thought.

Looking at time directly, inwardly, one sees that time is thought. It's not that time creates thought or that thought creates time; there is no difference. To see that is really extraordinary. To be in thought is always to be in time. You can watch the whole nature of thinking. You are either thinking about what has happened or what you want to happen or what might happen. To be in thought, is to be in time. To be in thought is to remove oneself from the actual livingness of now. To be either playing in the past or projecting into the future, both of which we do so much, is to be always removing oneself from

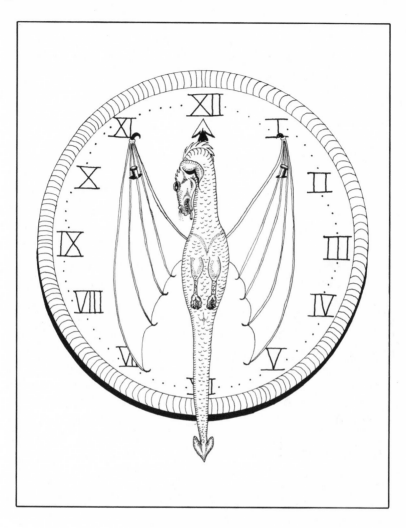

Memry is rather hung up

the ongoing reality of what is happening now. In this removal, which creates space between the experiencer and the experience, is time. Personality lives only in time. In the space between the seer and the seen, is time.

We talk about ecstasy, and what ecstasy really means is ex-stasis—being out of time. The ecstatic moments, those moments when there is no seer separate from the seen, are timeless. Thought is quiet in those moments. It is only when there can be a dying, an actual death of thought—which is death of personality, because thought lives in personality—that ecstasy comes. What I am is the accumulation of all my memories, thoughts. To be living in memories and the anticipations they foster, as most of us do, binds energy. I do not respond to the newness of life, to the immediacy of challenge because I am not there to do so; I am lost in time. When I am here, now, when this ecstasy occurs, there is energy unbound. To be alive with this tremendous energy is to be alive now. Actually, the present is all there is, for thought, being the past and the future, only occurs in the present. It's all happening now, which is a moment to moment thing. It is through thought—which continually generates time—that I remove myself from the actual living moment. Why do I do this? Again we go back to this whole thing of fear and pleasure. I do it because of pleasure, because time gives me pleasure. I get pleasure from thinking about the things I am going to do, remembering the things that I have done, thinking about the experiences I have had, and how rich and full my life may be or has been. You may see this in your own life if you look.

The playing in past or future, which is thought (which is time), removes you from that energy of the living moment. In that space between you and the living moment, time lives and with it sorrow. Yes, pleasure lives there too, but as we saw that is no different from sorrow. When one is removed from what is, which is to be in time, sorrow is there, though it, too, can be pleasurable. See how we drench ourselves in self-pity, the bittersweet quality of it . . . see it in yourself and then you will learn.

Of course one of the things one can do when one looks at time and sees the way of it, is to try and escape it. I say, "I want ecstasy" (but all I really want is a memory), or, "I want to be in 'the now,'" or I try to force out thoughts to stop time! Here obviously is ambition again, with fear. Everything we have been discussing together—pleasure, sorrow, belief—live in time. Violence itself is a product of time. As soon as there is a thinker trying to destroy thought (because there is an idea that to do it would bring more pleasure) the future crowds in. Most of us who become interested in the eternal—which, of course, is not in time—approach it through time, which is endless.

I'm not saying one should not be in time, or that it's bad, or that it does not have its appropriateness here and there in the scheme of living. Obviously I must remember my name; there are countless things in life where memory has a function and thought is useful. But thought has taken most of us over so that it becomes our totality; we live in time almost continually. What I'm talking about is a way of seeing, a way of being, where thought has no place. Thought comes mechanically out of memory, out of conditioning. The ideas we have about the way things are or should be come from conditioning. As soon as you have an idea about how something is or ought to be, then you are no longer looking at it or seeing it, and that includes seeing yourself. As soon as you say, "I know myself," you are only talking of the past, not what you are, but what you were. To believe that you know yourself is to be in time (the past), which removes you from inquiry, from seeing.

It may be comfortable, secure, to believe you know yourself. This comfort allays fear of future behavior that might destroy what we cherish from the past. To worship security as most of us do, is to live in time. As soon as you believe you know yourself, growth stops. The trick is to see it totally. This actually is what meditation is all about. To completely see my greed, my violence, my ambition, my fear, is a seeing that has its own movement. To see ambition as the psychological and spiritual danger that it is, is to move from it, a movement that does not occur in time.

As soon as I see the nature of time and try to make it go away, all I do is create it. That is part of the paradox of the bind of mind—whether we examine pleasure, freedom, time, or any other topic here, ultimately we reach a bind, a paradox, and anywhere we turn we're caught. It's possible to get a feel for the paradox, for the limitations of thought and the entire intellectual process.

I'm not expounding a philosophy, another system of thought, but rather what we are doing here together is using intelligence (not intellectual manipulation) in an extraordinary way. That is, we are using it to see itself, the seeing being a movement beyond imagined confines, and what is really important is not what I say, or agreeing or disagreeing. Seeing how mind works in yourself is the important thing.

Question. You mention boredom. Would you talk about it?
Answer. Nothing interests me. Nothing is worth doing. I'm restless, dissatisfied. I want excitement or change, yet there is nothing that seems worth doing. Of course, what I'm talking about could easily be seen as conflict. That's what boredom is—conflict. When I'm bored it's but an index there is conflict in my life. The world is always moving. There are walks to take, music, relationships, whatever. Sometimes there is boredom, sometimes not. Boredom is not external, it lives in you. Boredom is a freezing of movement, of energy, and when it happens it is interesting to observe what is occurring in oneself. See where the conflict lives. So often there are things one feels one has to do or should do, but really doesn't want to. When one looks for escapes (and that's what being bored is) one cannot even channel one's energy into escaping, for the mind still dwells (sometimes very quietly) on what you are trying to escape from.

The very young are not bored, at least not until they're programmed with "oughts" and "shoulds." When we are young, a day is long and full, a week is forever, a summertime an eternity. As we age time seems to accelerate; when we look back it's as if our life has flown by. Why is that? Why does psychological time, inward time, seem to go faster and faster? The young do not have the layering of conditioning that comes with aging. They do not live in thought so much. As aging comes thought increases, and time, which is thought, begins to fly. As adults, most of us live in thought so much. Our lives are so mechanical, so habit-bound, so automatic, that there is little actual living. So much of our lives are spent in time, which removes us from what may be called the "eternal." It is in this removal that time inwardly moves swiftly. You can also observe that when one is bored thought is very active. The more time one spends in time—which is thought—the faster time goes by.

Question. You say all there is is the present, and to live in it is to live. How can one not take into account the future when one does something? It seems undeniable to me that actions have their consequences. Some young people talk as if they can live

without the future—I cannot. From what I've seen, a total uncon-
cern for the future seems to create more problems than it solves.
Answer. First of all, it must be made very clear that I am not
saying that thought, and therefore time, has no place in living.
Obviously I must remember my name and countless other things.
Obviously I must consider the so-called future for many aspects of
living. All of this is very practical, very pragmatic. That actually is
where thought functions properly. (By "properly" I mean not
binding energy.) Thought is actually a practical tool. But for most of
us thought actually takes over and becomes us. Here a fragment of
the energy system takes over, tells itself it is of the utmost
importance, and through further fragmentation attempts to control
the remaining energy system of which it is but a part. The seeing of
this and the seeing of when thought is appropriate and when it is
not, is the business of awareness. What I am talking about is a way
of being in which thought is not appropriate.

Actions that seem to be done for future purposes are still only
done in the present; in a fundamental way the future is contained
in the present as is the past. In order to fly on an airplane I must
buy a ticket, but buying a ticket is buying a ticket; it is not flying
on an airplane. Buying a ticket *now* contains the seeing *now* that
if I am to fly on a plane I must have a ticket. Having the ticket
does not necessarily mean I will fly on the plane. Here thought
can operate very practically, remembering from the past that a
ticket is necessary to fly. The living activity of buying a ticket is
different. If one is busy in thought anticipating the flying either
with pleasure or fear or thinking of things that one will do upon
arrival, then energy is removed from the ticket-buying.

It is very popular among some groups these days to say that
what must be done is to live in the "now." The idea comes from
many sources: from interpretations of certain Eastern religions,
from certain fashionable "therapies," or whatever. There are all
kinds of ideas about just what living in the now means. It
becomes a desirable end, a sign that one is "in," or "high"; it becomes an ambition to be obtained. Confusion must come from the
ideas I have about living in the now. Out of the confusion and
conflict that ideas bring, one may try to make oneself "live in the
now," yet that is only another ambition. It is also possible to use the

idea of living in the now as an escape from responsibility—the ability to respond (real responsibility being the ability to respond totally to challenge). Under the guise of living in the now conflict in me can express itself as disorder in the world. I can feel superior to you who are caught in the "rat race." I can wallow in filth and disease and justify it by saying it's what's happening now. I can carelessly and casually impregnate someone because "now" is really all that matters. I can dull myself with drugs, since all that counts is immediate sensation. None of these has to do with the *timeless* seeing of what is, but rather are ideas about a preconceived state.

Question. What is "living in the now"?

Answer. Adventure. You never know what's going to happen. And it's dangerous because there is no security. Is there really any security? We are always trying to create it, but does it exist? The danger is there—the living is there. We turn away from it and pretend it isn't. You can walk down the street and be hit by a car. The earth can open up and swallow you. People run to find security—even the security of excitement. Everything gets old. Everything mechanical gets old—everything, no matter what it is. The strongest experience, the most powerful drug—it all becomes old. So the really exciting thing is to be living in the new, which can be just observing a bird on the wing, or the flicker of the light on a flower, or watching the way your mind works and how interesting it is to be the being that you are, which is always a changing being, a new being, a being who at every instant reflects the eternal, the timeless.

Question. Will you talk about worrying? I worry a lot and in listening to you it seems connected with time because I worry about the future. I also see that worrying about the future frightens me.

Answer. Obviously, worrying is one way fear displays itself. Fear as we saw lives only in time, in the future, out of the past. We are also afraid that should we not worry about the future, we would not get out of life what we want. Fear is the fuel most of us run on. Take away the fuel and what would move us? We are literally afraid of not being afraid. We have looked at this previously and asked whether fear is necessary for movement, for living; and we have seen how fear removes the energy necessary for response-ability.

Why worry? Why do we spend so many moments of our daily living creating the tensions and binds (psychological and physiological) that worry brings? Why do I spend so many of my living moments creating pain for myself? It is really important to see that it is I who do it to myself.

Worrying, which actually is pain, is one of the easiest ways of feeding personality, of not dying in the psychological sense. Worrying comes out of memory. The memory deposit lives in the cells, and its physiological aspect is expressed as tensions and tightnesses in the body. The feel of these tensions—again out of memory—become familiar and we call that feeling tone "me." To continually feed these tensions is to keep "me" intact. Worrying does it quite nicely. Pain turns into one of the great pleasures as it makes the self, or "ego," feel secure. Worrying gives the illusion of the continuity of the "I." I worry out of what I was to what I will be. Thought expressed as worry assumes that the "I" involved is the same entity. One of the by-products of doing Hatha Yoga is the de-conditioning of memory deposits in the body.

Thought, in fear, creates time, actually is time; and this sense of continuity, which is the movement of a being through time, is personality or the "I." It is in the "I" that pleasure lives always seeking the gilded cage of security of the known. I worry so much because it gives me great pleasure to do so.

Question. The seeing or awareness that you talk of seems so fleeting! I feel I have had moments of it, but it doesn't last. I also understand the impossibility of trying to hold on to it. I see too that the ambition to get more awareness or to have it all the time is futile. Yet in myself I feel pushed to do something. I have tried being quiet and just observing, but I realize I am trying with a goal in mind. I am not asking you what to do, but rather would like you to comment on what I've been saying.

Answer. The fact that "awareness" can become another goal to achieve and is therefore merely a word, is undeniable. Living awareness does not occur in time, therefore one cannot have it all of the time. In fact, one cannot have it any of the time for if there is a "me" having "it," then there is no awareness. Memory, where the "I" lives, can turn that energy of seeing into a pleasure and enjoy the image of being aware. This of course dulls you, for as soon as you operate out of any image there is no awareness.

When one gets involved in this type of inquiry, it's easy to become concerned with ideas about awareness. Real discipline does not concern itself with how aware I am or when I am aware. For when there is awareness, it just is. The trick is to discover when you are not aware; to see clearly you are not clear. The seeing that does not ask to be clear moves you so that clarity may come.

CHAPTER 7

ANALYSIS AND THE UNCONSCIOUS

In discussing analysis let us not concern ourselves with the different types of analysis, but rather how analysis by its very nature must work. Analysis of any type, be it Freudian, Jungian, or some other, has certain similarities in focus and mode of inquiry. Analytical jargon is very popular these days and has entered the common, lay language and has therefore suffused our consciousness: neurosis, psychosis, compulsions, anxieties, hangups, unconscious—words like these come up constantly. The very thinking in these terms is a form of conditioning that can easily create the symptoms the works talk about.

The analytical schools have told us that the way to get to know ourselves is through some form of analysis, in which the mind carefully goes back into memory and attempts to peel the layers of the onion of our conditioning to try to get at the very core of being that is the real me. All types of analysis work in this fashion—slowly through time we try to peel away the conditioning of memory, old things, things that have happened to us—all in an effort to know ourselves better.

Analysis plays in time. You go back through memory to find out about yourself. What self is it you are trying to find out about? A self that obviously has happened, has lived in memory, old traumas, old conditioning—one's old self. As this is happening what is going on? I am living, am I not? I'm going through life. I'm continually moving. Life is movement. As I go back and peel the onion, the whole process of living, which is itself conditioning, is going on and the onion is being continually reformed; analysis is endless. You

65

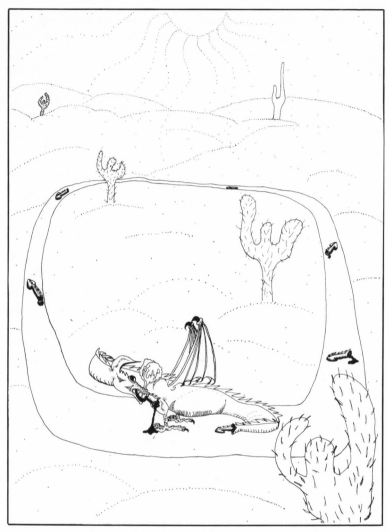

Memry on the endless path to know where

can spend a lifetime at it, because you are always playing in the past, in thought, in memory.

You spend years and years in the analytical game, and analysis itself can become a form of conditioning. You become very good at saying the words, or you become very good at telling yourself what's wrong with you, or telling others what's wrong with them.

Yet it doesn't seem to do anything. In fact, you can use the conditioning of analysis to justify your behavior: I do this or that because I have a phobia, or a compulsion, and, of course, you begin to use the analytical structure as a way of getting attention, and as a way of going to somebody and laying your responsibility on his shoulders, which is absurd, of course, because he can't respond for you—no one can.

Analysis has a lot of pleasure in it. I get wrapped up in myself, in all of my problems, and I try to work them out slowly through time—time, of course, being thought. But slowly through time (I can't do this too fast because I'm afraid of any real change), in 5, 10, or 20 years maybe I'll be all right and in the process I can keep myself very busy. If any of you have ever played in analysis there are some interesting things that happen. You may go back and relive a traumatic experience in memory and say, "Aha, here it is, I've got it." A week later you go back and you find that the thing you relived, the experience where you said, "Aha, now my whole behavior, my whole self is clear to me," you find it was only a fantasy that the mind threw up to keep you away from the real thing. And then you can go back a week later and find that this too has shifted because you are dealing with mind. Memory is sand. You just can never get it. It's always shifting, always changing.

Question.   Do you think that analysis is valueless?

Answer.   The problem you have is now. Analysis removes you from what's happening now and takes you back to what happened, what was. The very nature of it is such that it never solves the problem. It may give you certain insights; it may give you a lot of pleasure, but the problems just don't go away. Or if they do, new ones come and take their place. The symptoms may go away, but then another one comes out. The question is, can I cut through this whole thing? Analysis may take care of a specific symptom, but since the living problem is not gotten at, another symptom re-emerges. We may go from symptom to symptom until we find one that either we or society can tolerate.

You asked if analysis is valueless. It may be a door by which you begin to inquire about yourself and it may give you some fragmentary insights into yourself. If one who enters the door of analysis sees its nature and limitations and in the seeing moves from it—that is one thing. It is so easy to stay trapped in it, in the pleasure, the attention, the escape of it. For analysis easily becomes just another form of escaping from oneself. The thing about real problems is that they live here and now. The problem may have its roots in past conditioning, but it's not created by past conditioning. Let me give you an example of something I was involved with intimately:

There was a time when I was a very bad stutterer. I was trained in different analytical structures and began to use them to try to find out what stuttering was all about. I went back and relived traumas and found out to my satisfaction what initially brought about my stuttering. I began stuttering when my sister was born; I was seven years old. She took away much of the attention I felt was rightfully mine. Too, I hated her because she was interfering with my whole scene and when you're seven it's not nice or respectable to hate your sister. Therefore I held it in, and hid it both from the world and myself. I hated my parents because they had had her in the first place, and because they gave her a lot of attention. When people came over I was no longer the center; my sister was. There was great violence in me. Stuttering was an expression of the violence, and it served a number of purposes. I used stuttering as vengeance. It really upset my parents, which gave me much pleasure. And I used stuttering to reclaim attention.

I saw all this through the analytical procedure. I saw it very clearly. Then I waited for catharsis, the cure, the release from stuttering. It didn't come. I still stuttered. Learning the original reason for my stuttering didn't seem to make any difference. I began to ask myself why I was stuttering now. I don't hate my sister or parents now. I can even relive the hate and go through the whole cathartic thing and the hate is not there now. Yet still I stutter. Why?

I found out that the stuttering itself had become a useful tool to make myself feel special; it had nothing at all to do with my sister. And I used it to keep away from things I didn't want to do. In school I didn't have to prepare lessons because they would never call on me, a stutterer. And I was very up-tight around girls as a young man; I used stuttering as an excuse not to ask them to go out with me. I used it as a way of standing out in relationships—you remembered me. When you talk to a stutterer how do you feel? Uncomfortable, don't you? You try to pretend to the stutterer that nothing unusual is going on. You also give the stutterer special attention. You don't want to hurt his feelings. The stutterer, by stuttering, can actually control you.

Have any of you ever been around a seriously disturbed person? One who is called crazy, psychotic, schizophrenic? There is one thing they all have in common—their mere presence makes it almost impossible for you to attend to anything else but them. They totally dominate the scene. All so-called behavioral aberrations can be looked at in terms of how they control their environment and just what the person is getting out of it.

I was able to use stuttering to make myself feel unique, special, superior. (I stutter because my mind works too fast for my mouth!) It was also a way of operating in the world that always gave me an easy out. The fundamental fact was that I stuttered not because I hated my sister, but because it gave me dominance, attention, convenient excuses—in short, because it gave me pleasure. Of course, it contained in it pain and sorrow as pleasure does.

I found that out but my stuttering continued. Then I saw the reason I still stuttered was that it continued to give me pleasure to do so. I stopped stuttering when it became more important to me to communicate with people than to control them. It wasn't analysis or analytical insights that stopped the stuttering. It was the day-to-day seeing of just what stuttering was doing—in the doing of it. When you have a problem the problem displays itself in a living relationship. How the problem structures the environment happens at its occurrence, not 5 years or 8 years or 28 years ago, or when the initial reason for it was happening. Through analysis you can go back and find out all kinds of reasons for anything. The reasons for the onset of a behavioral problem are not why the problem displays itself now.

If you're involved in an analytical procedure, look into it and see what's going on. See what you're getting out of it.

Question.   Haven't you had insights through analysis?

Answer. Insights can come through analysis. But with my stuttering, for example, they did not matter at all. One can get limited, fragmentary insights through analysis, but because they deal only with the past they don't bring forth real change. Actually, one very useful insight that one may get through analysis is seeing its limitation. To see that is to see, and a movement comes from that seeing.

One might ask whether analysis is necessary before one could move from it. It was necessary only insofar as I felt that was the way to explore things. I felt that way because that was what I knew. I was conditioned to analysis. That does not mean it's necessary for anyone else to go that route.

I began to stop stuttering when I began talking to people. What happened is that I began teaching. When I began teaching I stuttered. Communication was important to me and stuttering interfered with communication. I'm not saying this is the way to stop stuttering. I'm saying that for me it became important to communicate. Stuttering was a side trip; it became tiresome. I had played with it a long time. Seeing its nature and how it interfered with communication was a movement from it.

I'm not offering this as a therapeutic technique. I'm simply offering it as a way of looking at the whole business of analysis; analysis is not necessarily the answer. To know something analytically doesn't make any real difference.

Question. Did you undergo any process to rid yourself of stuttering?

Answer. No. There was nothing cognitive or rational that way. It just began to leave me as I began to talk. It became a real hindrance, and I began not to need it anymore. It began to offer less. It was not the function of a flash, or a new insight, or anything like that. It was just the day-to-day living with it and seeing how it worked, what it was actually doing that made it more difficult to do. I only gave that as an example of knowing something quite well analytically and its persisting in behavior. When we do something, even out of the deepest conditioning, we get feedback. Actually we carry in us the sum total of our conditioning every moment, and every moment it displays itself for it is what we are. To see it totally is to see ourselves totally, and here, too. the seeing is a movement. You can see what you are doing now. Of course, it's very convenient to blame the past, your father and mother, all the circumstances that made you what you are today. But what you are today is now, and what you are doing is feeding yourself back now. It's you who are doing it—no one else. In terms of one's presumed psychological problems, the question to ask oneself is, "What am I getting out of them right now?"

Let's look at the unconscious, which has a great deal to do with what we've been talking about.

I have divided my mind into the conscious and the unconscious. The conscious mind is by definition the mind I have access to; either it is happening now, or I have access to it. The unconscious mind is the part of my conditioning that by definition I do not have access to, or only limited access. If I could get at it, it wouldn't be unconscious. This isn't complicated, it is quite simple.

I say, "If I could only get into my unconscious mind and find the real me." It could be full of bad things, or maybe it's full of good things. So I'm always flirting with mind. I can see the nature of thought—how competitive, how comparative it is, how it is always comparing me to you. I only know I'm good if I am better than you. I only know if the things I do are worthwhile on a comparative scale, and this is mind—very comparative. I say I want to get into the unconscious mind, get into myself in depth, find the real me. I put all kinds of hopes and fears into the unconscious, then flirt with it. But what makes one think the unconscious mind is any less petty, less trivial, less illusory than the conscious mind?

Why does one have an unconscious at all? When I hide something from myself, who is doing the hiding? If there is something in myself I don't want to see, how do I know I don't want to see it? Don't I have to know what's there in order not to want to see it? What I'm saying is, who is making it unconscious? Obviously I am—nobody else is, there is nobody else around—just me. If I'm making it unconscious, don't I have to know somewhere that here is something I just don't want to look at? The whole conscious/unconscious split is a huge game of peek-a-boo that I create to keep away from myself. It takes such extraordinary energy for me to hide myself from myself. These things come out through word games, through dreams, other devices; the unconscious is always bubbling out. It takes extraordinary energy to keep it down. Who's keeping it down? Obviously I am. Why? I must know there are certain things I don't want to see. Since I know I don't want to see them I must know just what they are. Why else feed energy into a construct that fragments me? That is what I mean by playing peek-a-boo. There is both a hiding from oneself and a pretense in hiding that one is not hiding at all.

The unconscious is thought that hides from itself. There are elements of myself that I don't want to look at. I don't want to look at my greed, my fears, my ambitions. I don't want to look at many of the things that make me the animal that I am (my violence, my uncaringness). I take these things that don't match the image that I have of what I should be, and I don't look at them. But in order for me not to look at them I must know they are there. So I put tremendous energy into creating the conscious/unconscious split.

But that is too simple. All of the learned men have written very thick books giving us very complicated methodologies on how to attack this serious, knotty problem. In doing so they have strengthened the game of dividing myself.

The question is whether it's possible to do away with the split, and not through analysis, which takes time. The endless process of analysis actually feeds fragmentation. Is it possible for intelligence, which is far more than mere thought, to instantly cut the knot of analysis, and see the nature of the division in oneself? It's a question to ask yourself, and the answer comes from delving into the problems yourself during the course of living. The only person who can open up these doors for you is you. And the only way to do it is to observe exactly what you are, not what you want to be, not what the experts tell you you ought to be, but what you are— now, because that's all there is. There is nothing else.

Question. Are there any drugs that lead to the unconscious?
Answer. There are drugs that blow one's controls so that the energy spent in hiding from oneself is momentarily lost. Ultimately, however, because the mind is stronger than these drugs and becomes familiar with them, it locks up again. The

mind can and does eventually wrap around the drug and incorporate it into its framework in not too long a time—I'm talking about even the most potent drugs around.

Question. Are dreams similar to the unconscious?

Answer. Dreams are complex. There are times when they could be called leakages from the unconscious. There are times when they are working over memory. Sometimes they just involve a stimulus cue. For example, an alarm goes off and an elaborate dream is made up to fit it. Because time is quite different in this state, something that may appear to take hours may take seconds in a dream. Dreams may express forbidden desires. They are creations of mind; most dreams are expressions of what ordinarily we don't look at. It's not that we can't; it's just that we don't ordinarily, because they involve an uncomfortableness. To dream is also a way of holding on to personality even in sleep. Dreaming ensures that I do not die, that the *me* is still around.

Let's look at dreams with regard to sexuality. A characteristic of being an animal (and that's what we are) is to be sexual. The attractions of the world are just there, yet there are sanctions, permissivenesses or unpermissivenesses in terms of who or what we can be attracted to. In many instances dreams express forbidden attraction—sometimes very symbolically. I may find him or her very attractive, but I have a secure relationship that could be destroyed by this other relationship. So there's conflict; I turn off. As we move through the world that's what we mostly do—turn ourselves off. It's very difficult to really look at another human being. He or she may attract you, then what are you going to do? It causes great difficulty. You run—in your mind.

Why do you analyze your dreams? Isn't it true that you're not analyzing the dream, but the memory of the dream? The dream itself is an expression, with feelings and overtones. As you go back and work it over, it changes and turns. It's like sand because you're not dealing with the occurrence. You're dealing with memory, which is always different. When you're doing that, the very act of doing it can remove you. The dream itself may be a release or an expression of something. To get involved with the dream is to be involved in memory. The memory may not necessarily be at all like the dream. When you are involved in this you are involved in sand—shifting—you can never get hold of it because nothing is there. It's all memory—mind.

Question. I think I heard you say that analysis conditions you. Would you go into that a bit more?

Answer. There's a magic to words, a power to them. Words so easily achieve a life of their own even if they refer to nothing. If I structure my behavior with words (and of course to structure it at all is to do so with words) I so easily find myself behaving within the confines of the very structure I set up. A structure that is initially proposed as an explanation of certain behaviors may for various reasons become popular. Then it turns into a belief. Once a structure becomes belief, the words take on life and dictate behavior to feed the belief. That is conditioning. The words "neurosis," "psychosis," "unconscious" have become very popular. They are part of everyday talk. To think of oneself or of another as neurotic is to feed behavior. One says, "It's not me. It's my neurosis," and fragmentation occurs.

Question. Don't you think the terms came into being because they described something that was really happening?

Answer. Of course that's the way some structures originate. I'm not saying it's incorrect to call an action neurotic or psychotic. I'm saying the words themselves take on a life that brings about the very thing they purport to explain. Here is the magic of words: they contain within them a self-fulfilling prophecy. What in-sanity actually is, is operating toward symbols as if they are real. It is interesting to see how much of what is called *society* is just this.

Chapter 8

IMAGES

Much of what is called living is playing in memory, which is playing in the past and the future, playing with ambition and fear. So much of what I see is through a veil of images. When I look at you it's very difficult to see you. You flatter me or you insult me. If you flatter me, I like it. Even if I know you are flattering me and disapprove of it, secretly I like it. You insult me and I don't like it. When I approach you again I see you through the memory of flattery and/or insult, so I'm not in touch with you the living person, but rather with a memory of what you were. I approach you and I respond to you out of that memory, which triggers response mechanisms in you, who have images of me. That is what's called relationship, which actually isn't real relationship at all, but rather images posturing in front of one another. When I relate to you through an image I have of you it is not you I am actually relating to, but rather with my own thoughts.

We have seen that in order to learn one must do away with all outside authority. There are so many outside authorities, and if one goes from one authority to another, then one never learns anything at all. You may learn to repeat what others have said, and you may learn to sound very clever, but you don't really learn. There is an authority that is even more difficult to do away with, that's more insidious, that has a much greater pull, and that is the authority of our own experience, our past, the authority of our memory.

I look at you; you have hurt me, or insulted me, been mean and nasty to me. It is so difficult for me to forget this when I see

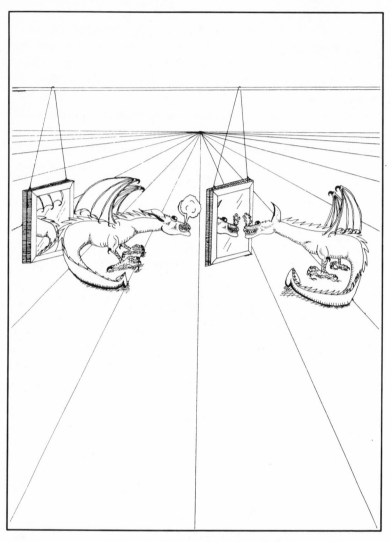

Memry relates only with himself

you now, so I approach you with memory, and of course, you do
the same to me. There isn't any relationship here at all, because I'm
not actually in contact with you. What I'm in contact with are
products of my own thought, my memories of what you were and
how you were with me—if you pleased or displeased me.

In my relationship with you, there are also expectations—what I want from you. I want company, or satisfaction, or love, so when I approach you I approach you out of my wants. When approaching you out of memory and desire, it is very difficult to see you as you are.

The whole of our conditioning is such that we approach one another out of images (memory and expectation), so we develop reciprocal trade agreements with one another. It's very difficult for me to be in contact with you because, really, I don't want you to change; I don't want you to be new. I want you to be the same so that I will know you, so that you are familiar and I can be secure in our relationship, whatever our relationship is. So fear is here. And, of course, you do this to me, too.

One of the things we're afraid of is loneliness. Out of the fear of loneliness I cling to relationship, yet there is no real relationship in fear, for what I cling to is the security of memory, which isn't relationship at all. Great loneliness comes from it, because out of the fear of being lonely and out of the demands I make on you out of the fear of being lonely, I cut off real relationship, which, paradoxically, produces more loneliness.

You know, it is only when I can be alone, really alone with myself, that real relationship is possible; only when I ask nothing of you can I be in real relationship with you. It is from this center of aloneness that true relationship comes. Loneliness and being alone are different things and unless one can be alone, one is forever lonely. Observe this in yourself.

I see how thought shadows and removes me from the living moment, which is all there really is. I see how thought incrusts image upon image. The older I get the more incrusted I am, and the more habits I have. That's why I stiffen. It's all habit—habit in the mind and habit in the body.

I see how much of what I call living is actually image, so I look for something beyond the image, something behind it. I look for the entity that is actually creating or spinning out the images. Where is it? I want to be in touch with the real being behind all of the spinnings of mind. So I look for the image-maker in myself. I see how so much of what is called living is actually being in image in the past, and upon seeing this the mind looks to see where it's coming from. I see how so much of what I call living is being in thought, how thought actually removes me from living, how thought is time, and that to be in time is sorrow. So I look for something behind this. I look for the thinker that is doing it. I have the image or images, and I look for an image-maker. I see thought and I begin to look for the creator of thought, the something behind thought—the thinker. It's very similar to the hunt in the unconscious for the real me, the pure and pristine entity that's not subject to the fluctuations of living.

So many of us are always searching to get in touch with ourselves, looking for the real behind the illusion. If I look very carefully at the split between the image and the image-maker, between the thinker and the thoughts, I find that the whole idea of the thinker is just another product of thought. There is no thinker; there is just thought. There is no image-maker; there are just images. If I want to learn about myself, actually learn about what I am and how I work, then I must look at the images, the thoughts, and see how they work. To look for something behind this because what I see appalls or dismays me, then I'm involved again in thought. I'm asking for something to be other than what is. If I say that I'm going to do away with images or thought, it simply becomes another thought or image, so I'm trapped again in the paradox, in the bind of mind which is always wrapping round me. To see this, to see how mind fragments, how I'm always looking for the thinker, for the maker of images, and how it is thought doing this, is to get in touch with the nature of mind and oneself.

Question. How can one escape one's past, what you call the building of images? It just doesn't seem possible. Have you managed it?

Answer. If I told you that it's possible and that I've escaped my past, you would either believe me or not, which would build an image of me in you, either of someone who is deluding himself or of a very special person. Either way inquiry is cut off. It doesn't matter what I am. If I'm a living example of the words does not matter. It is only when you can see for yourself what is possible that a movement may come.

One cannot escape the past in the sense of trying to run away from it. That is just the past trying to escape from itself. The mind is very sly; it can build the image of not having any images at all and seek that as an escape. Actually that's what many people who practice what they call meditation do. That, too, is just more play in image.

In observing the whole play of thought, of image, so there is no gap or space between the seer and what is seen, to see clearly that I am my images so there is no separation, for the separation itself is but image—to see that is to see. From the seeing, which is itself a stillness, a movement comes. Again, the seeing is the movement, which can never be asked for, never sought or demanded. As soon as there's an asker, a seeker, there's the separation between seeker and sought. If I am asking images to leave or seeking quietness, I can observe my ambition and that too is a seeing with its own movement.

CHAPTER 9

LOVE

Almost everybody eagerly seeks love and when it comes we try to hold on to it. We have many ideas about what love means, and the word *love* is used many ways. We are told to love our country, and that means that in the name of love, if we are young men, we go out and kill human beings we don't personally know—or be killed. If we don't, then we don't properly love our country. Religions tell us to love God and spell out how to do it in particular ways. If we love God, God will reward us for being good, for loving him properly, if not in this world, in the next—usually in the next. If we do not love God properly, God will punish us for not being good. Here the word *love* is used as reward and punishment, ambition and fear.

Ordinarily, when the word love is used it involves a demand, some type of reciprocal behavior. I say I love you, which means I expect attention from you. If you give me attention, well and good. If you don't, if you look at another person, I become jealous; so love has its opposite—hate. We are often told that love and hate are opposites. If you are my child and I love you, that means I expect certain kinds of behavior from you. If I don't get it, I generally withhold my love. The same is true with my friends and in other relationships. Ordinarily when we look at the word love, it involves a demand, a payment. It's like a reciprocal trade agreement; if you look, you can see it in relationship. You do this and that for me, then I'll satisfy you with company, sex, and so forth. That's how what we generally call love works.

Let's ask ourselves, seriously, if love can ever make any demands at all and still be love. If I make a demand and call it

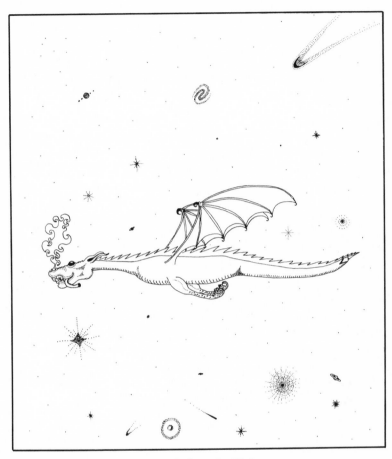

Memry adrift in the Universe

love, what am I actually interested in? I'm interested in my pleasure, my experience, my intensity—myself. If I'm doing that, am I loving you? Can love, if there is such a thing as love, make any demands at all and still be love? If it makes a demand, why sanctify it or call it by a name like love? Why not call it what it actually is—pleasure? If I say I love you and I expect you to be any other way than you actually are, am I loving you, or am I just involved again with expectation or demand? If I say I love you and I'm asking you to be different or to respond to me in a certain kind of way, am I loving you? Can love have an opposite?

If you do something I don't like, I hate you or become jealous. Is that what love is all about? If I love you when you please me and hate you when you don't, what am I involved with—you or my pleasure? Can love make demands and still be love? As soon as there's a demand, an expectation, a want, then I'm no longer actually relating with you—now. Again, I'm relating with image, in thought, in time, because expectation always has a future to it; I'm not actually relating with you at all.

Is there a way of being that may properly be called love, that makes no demands? Is there a meaningful way of being that may be called love that does not involve pleasure? If there is, how do I get it? I think I want it. How do I cultivate it? When love comes into my life, the rush of it, the bloom of it is a tremendous energy. When it leaves, I look for it again. I want to cultivate it. I want to keep it by my side always. I want to ensure that it will be with me tomorrow and next year.

Love is not a hothouse flower. If you try to cultivate love, it dies. You can go and pick a daisy in a field, and it's lovely and you bring it into your house and put it in a glass of water, but it dies. Love is wild, too. It does not live under cultivation. It lives only in the wild—only in freedom. The more I grab onto love, which is actually grabbing onto memory, the more it eludes me.

Most of what is called love contains enormous fear. In our relationship if I need you, and call that love, I then fear you will leave me or die. I'm afraid I might leave you or that my love is dimming or any of the countless fears that go on in a so-called love relationship. If there's fear, then of course ambition and demand are there, too. Love never blooms where there is fear. You can watch it in yourself. As soon as ambition, the holding on, comes in, love flies away. Real love breeds no fear, has no opposite. It just is an energy in relationship. As I grow older, because of my habits and demands, my fear of loneliness, I demand love even more and love becomes more difficult. I settle into convenient, comfortable relationships that put love very far away. As I get older and more inflexible, love becomes only a memory.

When does love come? In order for me to love you, to actually be in a relationship that may be called love, I must see you as you actually are, otherwise I'm not in touch with you. In order to see you, of course, the vehicle of seeing must be clear; the lens must be clean. In other words, I must see myself. When the gap or the space between the seer and the seen is not there, when, in fact, time, which lives only in the space between the seer and the seen, is not there, then love may flower. When there is a quietness so that I may see you (because I can only see you when I'm not asking for anything from you, and I can only not ask something from you when there is quietness in me), it is only then that real relationship grows. It is only then that love may come. It may not come; it comes and goes on its own. To ask for it is to ensure that it doesn't come.

Love itself is a blessing, a benediction, and the blessing of love, which is a renewal, comes only when there is an innocence that puts away all hopes and expectations, all flatteries and insults, all memories. It comes only when there is a stillness so that I may see you. Love is not a holdable commodity, which one puts in a box to keep, then takes out at appropriate times. Love comes and goes. Either it's here or it's not. If it's not, it's not; if it is, it is. The idea, like many others in this book, is so simple most people completely miss it.

What am I to do? I want love, yet the more I try to seek it—which is seeking a memory, seeking pleasure—the less I have of it. When I try to hold and secure love, to put it safely in a box, it dies. What can I do? All one can do is leave open a window so the breeze of love, the freshness and newness of it, may come in. If a window is open, the breeze may still not blow in; there is no guarantee. There is, however, one guarantee: if the window is not open, the breeze will not blow in.

The opening of the window is getting to know oneself—seeing clearly the nature of the being one is. For only if there's clarity in me can I see you, see the livingness that is you. That's what real meditation is all about. Meditation as we shall see is involved with clearing the lens.

Question. Is it making a demand when you see your loved one harming himself? You are concerned only because you love him.
Answer. I might be in direct relationship with you and love might bloom in that relationship. Part of what I see is a being doing self-destructive things. That doesn't interfere with love. It does interfere with love when I want to change you. Here is a

being destroying himself. In some ways the whole process of living is destruction. What am I really concerned about? What's the problem? Is the problem really concern about a being destroying himself? It's all right to be concerned. That isn't putting a demand on the being, is it? But if in the name of concern you try to make someone change to fit an idea that you have of what the person ought to be, that is different: then you lose touch with the person. If you look closely at the idea or image that you have of how the person should be, you will see it involves self-gratification. The change you envision would lighten your life, bring it more pleasure, or something similar.

Say there's relationship with a being taking drugs. It's not that you love a being whom you would love better were he not taking drugs. That is just a play in mind, because love doesn't work that way. It is a very difficult thing to allow someone just to be—very difficult. But isn't that something you want for yourself—just to be allowed to run your own changes in life? Concern may be there, but concern has nothing to do with the fact that I'm demanding anything of you. That's different. Concern can be like care. Real care and love are not different.

The fact is I do make demands. I do have certain expectations in relationship. The really interesting thing is not to try to change this, but rather to see exactly how expectations affect your relationships, how demand destroys real relationship; you can only see it when you are doing it. I have heard people say, "Does that mean I have to give up my family, since there isn't any real love there, and I should remove myself?" It doesn't mean that at all. If I see how my life is full of demands and how they remove me from you, from creative living, if I observe how the whole thing works, the seeing itself brings forth a movement. If I try to change my relationship out of effort, whether it be to leave or stay, conflict increases and love does not bloom. As in the case of the tree falling, the seeing is a movement.

Most relationships are built around fear. Fear that you will leave me, or that I'll leave you, or that you'll die before me and I'll be lonely, or that we'll grow old and our relationship will change. You can see it in relationships. I'm afraid to allow myself to look at another human being because that human being may turn me on; if

I get into this relationship it may hurt the other relationship. There is always that conflict—out of fear. To see it is really interesting because the seeing of it brings forth changes. The reality is that what I'm continually looking for—security in love—doesn't exist. There is no security. Tomorrow my husband or wife may leave me, my children may renounce me, a car might hit me. That's the reality of living.

Question. Then I guess we shouldn't love?
Answer. No. Ordinarily what we call love isn't love at all; it's fear and pleasure. Love only blooms when there's a forgetting of expectation. Love only lives when there's no fear. You cannot have fear and love together.

But there is fear, and if I try to get rid of it in order to get love, then all I get is more fear and conflict. So I begin to live with my fear. I learn to see it in my relationships, in how I move with my wife or my husband or my children. I listen to the sound of my voice, the demands I subtly make, the demands that are subtly made upon me. You can see it from moment to moment as you're living anywhere. It is there all the time. The demands are not only in the other person. They are in you. To see it is to learn about the nature of the animal that you are.

If you ask someone, "Do you love me?" do you believe the answer? You don't believe it. You're just asking for a programmed response. When somebody loves you, you know it. It is a living relationship. It is an energy. To be involved in seeking love is to be placing a demand on the other person, which immediately negates even the possibility of the thing itself.

The more we look for love to be there always, the more it's not there, because love comes and goes—in any relationship. We want love to last forever. "Forever" is an idea, a product of time. Forever does not exist, there is only now. Look at relationships, see what they are, which may permit love to come in. It may, but if you do not do it, then most assuredly love will not come.

When we're young and open there are times when love may come in a rush of energy. In the initial meeting there are not all of the incrusted habits, so there's newness, freshness. That is why many people spend their lives running from one lady to another, or one man to another, always looking for that flash of newness. You can go from one person to another and that, too, gets old. We expect the memories that we have of love to be the same each time. But we are different. When love comes in, it is a different thing, though love is love.

Love is timeless. It does not live in time. It does not live in the memories of the past or in anticipation of the future, but only in the living moment, in what may be called the eternal. Love only lives in death. Only if I can die to myself, to memory, to thought, to the past and to the future, only then may love come. Love lives when time dies.

One of the presumed wise men (we don't know if he was wise or not, we don't even know if he lived, and it doesn't matter) is reputed to have said, "You must be as a child." And that doesn't mean childish. Children have a quality of innocence, which comes from forgetting. You can insult a child and he'll forget. But if somebody insults you, you don't forget. If you don't forget, you can't love, because innocence is gone. Some of us try to put the child on a pedestal and say that we must be like children again. But we are not children. There's a difference between being childlike and childish. When we try to relive our old experiences, we are being childish, and by childish, I simply mean behaving in an inappropriate mode. When you call your children childish it means they are acting in an inappropriate mode for where they are. If you call your child of, say, nine-years-old, childish, that means he is acting like a three-year-old, which is very different from being childlike. To be an adult is different from being a child. It means seeing the nature of one's conditioning and how conditioning destroys innocence. In the young, love may come relatively easily because conditioning and habit have not taken hold. For adults it's not so easy because they are more incrusted with mind, thought, knowledge, and memory.

I am living with my husband or wife and I have an expectation in myself that I should love my husband or wife all the time and that he or she should love me all the time, that I should love my children all the time, and that they should love me all the time. But isn't that fantasy? Doesn't it create enormous conflict? Isn't it just another product of thought, another idea, another image? The concept or idea of *all the time* which plays such a large part in most of our lives does not exist outside of the mind creating it.

Question. Why do I feel guilt when I have bad thoughts about my husband?

Answer. What is guilt? Doesn't guilt only live when you aren't matching up to an image, when you aren't being the way you think you should be? And doesn't the demand that love live all the time automatically create guilt? Because obviously, it doesn't live all the time. So you aren't living up to your expectations and not only that, your presumed loved one isn't living up to your expectations of him, because he's not loving you all the time either, although he may be saying so continually. The word is not the thing and saying that you love is not the same as loving. That is the way of it. When there is love words are superficial. Love just is.

As we get older we get further and further away even from the expectation of love. We begin to wonder if there ever was such a thing as love because we are so engrossed in memory and demand. Any time there is expectation there is always fear. When there is fear there is never love—just habit. Habit is a turn-off: it removes me from seeing what is. I'm a creature of habit, which is a continual problem. You can never get away from yourself: you are the habits; the habits are not external to you.

Question. What is the relationship between love and responsibility?

Answer. What is responsibility? Ordinarily, the way the word *responsibility* is used means doing something I really don't want to do, but think I should—so there is no love there. What real responsibility is, is response-ability, the ability to respond to the living situation, which has nothing at all to do with obligation. Love is response and to be able to love is to have responsibility.

I have often been told that love, as discussed here, just isn't possible in ordinary relationships. How can I live that way? I have a family, friends. It's not possible to live totally without demand. Whether or not it is possible to live totally without demand is not the question. To say that I can or cannot is just an idea involving hope, expectation, and of course, fear. The question is not whether it is possible or not to have love all the time in ordinary relationship. See how ordinary relationship works and how demands stifle love, then, perhaps, from the seeing of it, one's ordinary relationship may have a movement that makes the relationship truly free, and love can only live in freedom. Freedom doesn't mean laissez-faire activity. Freedom means responsibility, which means the ability to respond always to the new in the other person, which means no demands.

In listening to the words of this person perhaps you may come to think one should live in relationship without demand. So I may say to you, "Demands destroy love; make no more demands on me and I'll make no more on you." To demand from you not to make demands on me is a demand. To demand from myself to cease making demands is a demand, too. A demand that lives in image and ambition creates enormous internal conflict. The trick is not to do away with demands, but to see how they work. The seeing is the movement.

To be free I must learn to live with myself. Until I can really live with myself I must put demands on you, which precludes love.

I've heard people ask about children. My children are very young, so I have a responsibility to take care of them. Seeing the child and seeing the situation the child is in, is its own response. Obviously a child needs care. That's part of the ability to respond to the situation, which is what real responsibility is. But ordinarily what we mean by responsibility is to try to make the child into some idea that we have of what the child ought to be—a good citizen, a creative intelligence, whatever we have in mind.

Real responsibility has no structures. Real response-ability doesn't move in fear. Real responsibility is a moment to moment thing. The expectations of relationship only kill real relationship.

Love is an energy, not a word. Love is an energy that lives in relationship, which seeks no return, has no opposite. Only that which makes demands or has expectations has an opposite, which is hate. If when you please me I love you, and when you don't please me I hate you or become jealous, is it you I'm involved with, or simply my own pleasures? That isn't love at all. Real love is its own benediction. Real love does not seek for anything outside itself. Real love lives only in silence. It does not live in thought because thought is always comparing and when you are comparing you are not loving.

CHAPTER 10

SEXUALITY

In these times of so-called sexual liberation, sex is coming out of the closet. Sexual mores are changing and there's much confusion in personal living about what is and is not appropriate. The old structures and taboos are breaking down, leaving in their wake confusion and conflicts. For most of us, sexuality, in one form or other, becomes an extraordinary problem. We want sexual relief. We worry about our sex lives, our adequacies or inadequacies, so that sexuality becomes a focal point of life, and a great problem.

If you're young the sexual conflicts are there because society says one thing about sex and does another. Your peers and friends say one thing, your parents another. The physiology makes its own demands. How is one to know what to do? Actually, the problem of sexuality is not divorced from the problems we've been discussing together—sexual binds are part of the binds of mind.

Real living always involves passion. By passion I mean an abandonment, a giving up of oneself. That is what real passion is. Sexuality of course is genetically programmed, it's part of the reproductive and evolutionary process and for this reason (though the reasons really don't matter), sexuality is one of the places where passion most easily occurs. For a moment, 5 seconds or whatever it is, I lose myself in you, in the passion of the sexual act. Since for the most of us it is only in sexuality that this passion usually lives, sexuality becomes extraordinarily important, and we hunger for it again. I worry if my orgasm is as adequate as hers, or his. Am I getting enough? Is it good enough? Is it deep enough, rich enough,

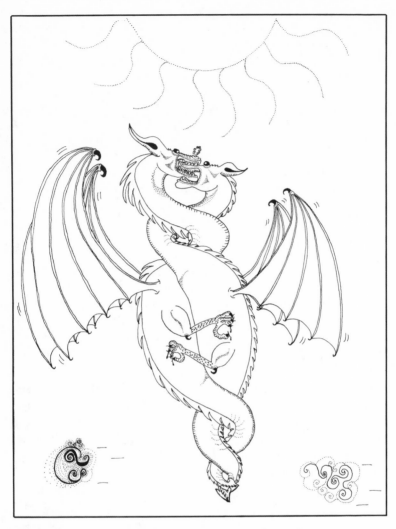

Will Memry's battle with sex be one?

will it be better, am I getting older, is my potency leaving me? How am I going to live with all of these sexual problems?

It seems as if I have hooked most of the passion of living into sexuality, and that's the real problem for most of us. If there were passion in living, in just day-to-day living, then sexuality wouldn't be the problem it is. It would just be something the animal does or does not do, depending upon its appropriateness. Knowing when sex is and isn't appropriate is the business of awareness. In fact, knowing how sexuality works and its appropriateness is movement into real adulthood.

The problem for most of us is there is no passion in living. For most of us, passion is an exclusive concomitant of copulation, so all of the problems of sexuality are, again, the problems of mind. Sexuality, as I think most of us approach it, contains in it all of the problems we've been looking at—a miniature universe that contains pleasure, fear, ambition, time, conflict. If in the act of sexuality itself one is looking for release, for orgasm, then the mind is in the future, in time. There is also the memory of past acts and anticipation of culmination, which is pleasure. The fear of not being satisfied or of not satisfying, involves ambition. As I am involved in this, which is fundamentally being involved with myself, with thought, I have removed myself from you, from the intimacy of living relationship.

Occasionally orgasm involves passion (abandonment), and I hunger for more of it. The hungering is the pleasure. Yet the more I seek it the more difficult it is to get. As I become older, it becomes more difficult to have freshness in sexuality.

When I'm occupied with sexuality I'm not actually occupied with being sexual; I'm looking for release. As I do that, I soon begin to fantasize in order to attempt to get more feeling. I remove myself from you. I play in fantasy, and so do you, so that really there aren't two people involved at all. Then sexuality is habit-bound and stale.

Much of what is called sexuality is used as a tranquilizer, a sedative, a way of turning oneself off. One can observe the fact that the actual thing one is looking for in sexuality, in orgasm, is release. What happens when release occurs? The extraordinary energy of sexuality is gone; you're turned off. So the very thing most of us seek in sexuality is to be turned off. The mind is always hungering for orgasm. But when orgasm comes energy leaves—it's blown. You can easily observe all of this in yourself.

If one is really involved in a true sexual relationship, orgasm is not important. It's sexuality itself that's important. The seeking of orgasm turns you off to what you're doing *now*. Instead of relating with another human being, we relate with our needs out of image. Most of the time we're relating to our own demands, and orgasm is used as a tranquilizer to cool ourselves out. I'm not saying this is bad or good—I am simply observing the way it works.

It is because sexuality is often approached as a tension and relaxation dance which blows enormous energy, and also very often removes you from the person you're dealing with, that many so-called spiritual or religious movements have attempted to negate sexuality in one way or another. Sexuality does potentially create conflict which binds energy, but any attempt to stop the conflict by eliminating or controlling sexuality only creates more and often greater conflicts. If you try to turn off your sexuality and go celibate because you think it's going to open up all kinds of spiritual doors for you, all you're doing is creating more pressures, more conflict, more tension. If you negate sexuality and become celibate out of ambition—which, of course, is a negation of what you are—the negation contains conflict. This is not to say that celibacy may not be appropriate to a particular life style.

Sexuality is an energy system and there are many ways to play within the system. Ordinary sexuality is one, celibacy another, and what is sometimes called Tantric Yoga is yet another. Tantric Yoga involves the holding back of orgasm so that energy is recycled instead of released.

In the process of getting to know oneself totally, the workings of one's sexuality are just there. To be an animal is to be sexual. (That is what we are—animals.) We fragment ourselves (actually it is thought that does this) into separate parts or centers—intellectual, emotional, sexual. A living organism is really not fragmentable, except in thought. Any time there's a total response in any situation, the whole being is there and because the being is sexual, sexuality is always there in any total response.

Most of us have isolated our sexuality into the genital area and consider sexuality to deal primarily with genital responses. But certainly genital responses are not appropriate with everyone. If I feel they are not right with you, I turn you off and consequently I turn myself off because I am no longer responding fully to you.

I walk down the street and I cannot allow myself to see you be-cause you might turn me on. Supposing you do, what am I going to do? I have my own relationships. I'm afraid of jeopardizing them, afraid of losing what I have or of getting involved in relationships built on secrecy. So ordinarily I cut off the world around me because I'm afraid of being turned on. I'm afraid of seeing you. I'm afraid of love because I don't know how to handle it. In this culture, perhaps in all cultures, but certainly for us, love and sexuality generally have a genital and copulatory orientation, so that if I allow myself to see you, to see your beauty and be turned on by it, then it begins to bring on all kinds of complications in my life. I don't know how to respond. I don't know what to do with the energy of being turned on. So I turn myself off, which also takes energy. To look at you brings complications, but not to look at you means I'm turning myself off. You know, it is endless. Human beings are constantly involved with one another. Anyone can be turned on by anybody else, not only between male and female, but also between members of the same sex. In fact, sexuality is polymorphous and by this I mean it can occur in any relationship—with an animal, a flower, the world itself.

Here is another area of great conflict. Society and my conditioning both have something to say about sexuality and the images I build of myself out of this conditioning make it very difficult for me to be open to you. If I am open to you things come in that are at times contrary to my image. So fear is here and out of fear I shut myself down and you out.

Question. You said that for most people sexuality is primarily genital and seemed to intimate there is some other way of operating sexually. Can you talk a little more about that?

Answer. In any total response, because we are sexual animals, there is sexuality. To have a free flow of energy, there must be sexuality. It may display itself in a look, a touch, in a quality of attention. If one is totally relating with anything—a flower, a musical instrument, a person—sexuality is there. The binding of energy in the genital area and the conflicts that arise from this, come out of conditioning. It is a seeing of this conditioning and how it works that brings forth movement. To see any conflict, including sexual conflict, is to bring movement. Yoga, in its different aspects, is an activity that deals directly with sexual energy, and plays with the movement of energy throughout the total system.

Question. What does sexuality have to do with love?
Answer. Love involves passion, an abandonment of oneself. It is an energy that lives only when there is death of personality. In the sexual act passion seems to come relatively easily. In a moment of passion love may come, though as sexuality itself becomes ritualized and habit-bound, passion leaves and is harder and harder to come by. We remember it was once there, and we seek it again. In seeking for an old experience to repeat itself, we turn away from newness. Love is always marked by a freshness, an innocence. When love is the total flow of energy, it contains sexual elements. Copulation can and oftentimes does occur without any love at all. It is often simply a self-centered activity where passion does not live.

Question. I am familiar with some of the problems you speak of and can relate to them. I know that I turn myself off with sexual conflict, but I did not hear you give any solutions. What can I do?
Answer. I think most of us want to be fed solutions to our problems. Solutions never come until the problem is clearly seen. When that happens the solution is just there: You don't have to look for it or create it; it's contained within the problem. The trick is to see the problem, not to look for the solution. Sexual conflicts are part of the total conflict of our lives. One can only see them clearly as one sees oneself totally. How rare it is to see anything without there being an entity that is seeing something external to itself. Have you ever looked at a flower and not called it a rose or a violet, not said it is blue or red, pretty or ugly, not compared it to some other flower? How unusual it is for this to happen! A flower is a relatively static thing. How much more unusual it is to see oneself in a nonfragmented way. Is it possible for a human being to see himself in an instant totally so that the seer is the seen? The seeing

does not occur in time. It is not introspection, which always plays in time. It is actually what real meditation is all about.

Question. A flower is outside of me. My mind is inside. Doesn't that make a difference?

Answer. Previously we talked about the internal and external and we saw how they actually are not different. Really to see a flower or oneself is not different. We can look at the so-called external more easily because seeing its nature does not open us to as much pain as seeing ourselves; we have a huge vested interest in our ideas about ourselves. Part of our self-image involves the creation of the external, for we do like something out there to feel better than.

Is sound or sight external or internal? For thousands of years philosophers have tried to answer this question with thought—to no avail. Actually sound has no locus, no point of reference, so thought cannot explain it. Sound is a product of living relationship that moves beyond the boundaries of the external and internal.

Most of us consider the skin and everything inside of it as the "me," or internal. Everything outside the skin is "not me," the external. Out of that structure, which we are conditioned to believe in, we fragment ourselves from the world, making it into "self" and "other." Living relationship, real communication, which is love, transcends those boundaries because there is no internal or external. The internal and external are not different at all. The world we create is but an expression of ourselves. If the world is violent, in turmoil, uncaring, it's because we are. There's really no difference at all between the internal and external. Communication that breaks the boundaries of all divisions is an energy that has sexuality within it. This energy is love.

CHAPTER 11

MEDITATION

Meditation is a fashionable word these days, and activities that are called meditation are prevalent and popular. Actually, to be on a "higher" path is a highly competitive activity. Spiritual competition is fundamentally no different than physical or material competition. In fact, spiritual competition because of its slyness, can become all-engrossing, because people cannot permit themselves to see what's involved. If you're a businessman, it's all right to be competitive and to recognize it as such. But if you're on a spiritual path, you're not supposed to be competitive; it's not nice, it's not spiritual.

To be hungering after spirituality is no different than to be hungering after anything else, though we usually place it on a higher plane. It's like trying to cultivate humility, which is very amusing. The greatest dominance games are played in the attempted cultivation of qualities like humility: I'm very humble, which means, of course, I'm better than you who aren't. True humility is never cultivated; it comes only when I see clearly that I'm no different from you, no better than anybody else. No matter how great my achievements are, no matter how externally significant I appear, the fact is I'm really no different than you in a very fundamental way. From that knowledge comes real humility. It comes from seeing yourself, but this cannot be cultivated.

In this day and age we are quite jaded. We go from "trip" to "trip," like drugs, sensitivity or awareness training, religious or spiritual groups; gestalt, encounter, psychodrama. We go from one to the other so that they are a part of us and we become very sophisticated. We've accumulated much experience, and out of all this

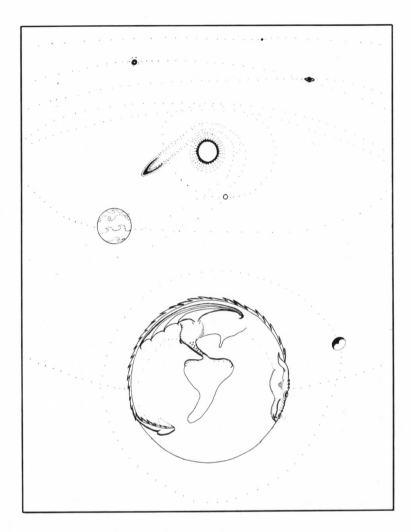

Memry loses himself

experience, which is conditioning, we approach meditation to add to our list of accomplishments. But what is it that we want? We move from one structure to another, from one form of stimulation to another, from one guru or master to another, always searching, thinking, seeking. Finally we come to meditation. Books, gurus, our friends paint extraordinary pictures of achievements possible through meditation. They say if we attain deep meditation we'll reach our heart's desire: serenity, bliss, eternal life, a better next lifetime, whatever.

There are many so-called meditative techniques, many yogas, many breathing exercises, mantras, repetitions of syllables, many mechanical ways of quieting the mind. Ordinarily these meditative techniques are always used as stepping stones. In other words, I meditate for something: to get into a higher state of consciousness or to quiet my mind. What is usually called meditation aims toward something else. That is ordinarily the way people look at and approach meditation. You can ask people if they meditate and they say, "Yes, I meditate! I quiet my mind. I'm trying to get in touch with this or that, or see this vision or that vision," and you know, it's possible. You can see any vision you want to see. If you want to see Christ or Krishna or Buddha, the mind can create them. It's really quite possible.

Is meditation ever a stepping stone to somewhere else? If it is, aren't we playing again in ambition? If I'm meditating to get somewhere else, am I not just involved in thought again? If I'm busily involved in trying to quiet myself, isn't that just what we're talking about—being lost in the bind of mind?

Look, I am very noisy. If I observe the nature of the noise, which is thought, I see just what we have been discussing together—a fear, ambition, belief, conflict. I see what a distraction the noise is, how much sorrow is in it. I say to myself—wouldn't it be nice to be still. So I try through effort to quiet myself. Yet a mind ambitious for quietness is a noisy, busy mind. Through one mechanical technique or other a temporary stillness may ensue, but the noise returns.

All mechanical meditative techniques are limited. It is possible mechanically to quiet your mind. You can say a word over and over again—"Om," "Hare Krishna," anything, it doesn't matter. You can say it and a quietness, which is a sedation will occur. Most of us use meditation to remove ourselves from the unpleasantness of living, so that what is called meditation is just another sedative. One can quiet the mind mechanically in all sorts of ways: do mantras over and over again, or chant, or breathe a certain way. You can take a tranquilizer, which is also mechanical. You can sit in front of a television and mechanically quiet your mind. Of course, some of these have a more esoteric feel to them than others, but they are all mechanical ways of quieting the mind. Those of you involved in these meditative techniques, if you observe carefully what you are doing I think you will find there is always a part of you holding back, watching and waiting for changes to take place, for the promises to be realized, for the *goodies* to happen, like smoking grass and waiting for it to come on.

The reason meditation of this sort is so popular is because people really want something mechanical that will change their state of consciousness. There are many things that can do it, but it's really very different than living awareness. Most of what goes on in the name of meditation is just another tranquilizer. It's a way of cooling oneself out, removing oneself from what is, removing oneself from seeing totally the living moment, which is eternal. For to see any living moment—totally—is to see that which is eternal. Unfortunately, what is usually called meditation is a way of removing oneself so that one gets lost in the projections of one's own mind. There may be a lot of pleasure there. If you sit and try to see visions, eventually you will, because the mind is infinitely facile in spinning out anything it wants to see. If you concentrate on anything long enough it will come to you. Concentration, which always involves effort, is not meditation. Concentration is a narrowing of the spectrum of awareness, a strengthening of thought, for it is thought that is doing it. In concentration there is always one who is concentrating—a separation that is thought. Real meditation is a widening of the spectrum of awareness that excludes nothing; there is never effort or force.

What are those meditative techniques all about? If you have a child and the child is noisy, and you give the child a toy, the toy will absorb him; the child will become quiet in the toy. When you take the toy from the child, the child becomes noisy again. When the toy becomes old and shoddy, the child then cries out for a new toy and becomes noisy again. The same is true of meditative techniques; they are all toys. Their real use, if given with awareness, is that one does them until one sees their limitations and then the seeing of the limitations of any mechanical device, of any structure, is its own freedom. Let's look into this more deeply.

Let's look at Zen as a meditative toy. You go to a Zen master. (Obviously any structure in which some members are called masters automatically sets up a dominance/submission relationship.) You go to a man versed in Zen and say, "Zen master, tell me all about myself. Tell me where it's at. Tell me what's happening?" Then the Zen master may do one of those charming, paradoxical things one reads about: hit you with a stick, tell you to listen to the sound of one hand clapping, or send you away on a Zen mission; when you return he'll do it again. Or he'll tell you to go sit with your face against the wall for an hour a day. Then he'll tell you to do it for two hours a day. Then you'll come back and he'll tell you to do it for three hours a day—so say Zen stories.

Why does the Zen master, when you come to him with a question of great intensity, laugh at you or hit you with a stick? Why does he do any of the quixotic things the people in these Zen stories do? What is he saying to you? The answer isn't complicated, really. He's telling you of the absurdity of your coming to him and asking him questions that one can only answer by looking within oneself. Of course you keep coming back until you see the absurdity yourself, then you don't come back. But why doesn't he just tell you this directly? Why doesn't he just say, "Look, that's nowhere. No other human being can answer your question for you. You've got to find out for yourself." Why doesn't he just say that? Because he knows you are not going to believe him, that you're just going to go to someone else who is going to tell you what you want to hear. And when you do that, you're lost. So at least if you keep going back to him, maybe you'll have a chance. And that, essentially, is the game of Zen.

Once there was time for that sort of thing, but now there's no time. The years spent on heroic or spiritual quests are not the point. The challenges of today are so extraordinary there's no time for that sort of play.

In the past, every now and then an adult would emerge, look around, and see the childishness of people. Toys would be given to the children in the form of structures or rituals to keep them quiet (though it was a mechanical quietness) and out of trouble.

The toy was such that one could outgrow it by seeing its nature. Mantra, as a toy, may remove you from your usual conditioning, yet the doing of it contains all the problems of living. In mantra there's ambition and, of course, fear. Conflict is there as well as belief. Since it removes one for a time from the ordinary habits of one's life, it may be possible to see in mantra one's ambitions more readily. Yet mantra is double-edged because it, too, is conditioning, as are all mechanical things. The real use of any mechanical toy is to see the nature and limitations of the toy. The mechanical can only give you mechanical results; to see that is to move beyond the mechanical.

The time of our adolescence is ending. If the species is to answer the challenges, adulthood is necessary. Real meditation is not a toy. It actually is necessary. Real meditation involves the total revolution of one's being and is the font of a new evolutionary principle.

What then is real meditation. It is not a stepping stone to get somewhere else. Meditation is not a possession; it cannot be owned. It is not something that one does mechanically for a certain period of time. Real meditation is a way of living, of being, that is its own blessing, that asks for nothing outside itself. There is no way to practice it. People are so hung up in practices, like doing sums or multiplications so that they can have a possession. I'm going to meditate and get this possession that I call "enlightenment" or "samadi," then I'll have it and be able to display it to my friends.

Real meditation is not something one does for five minutes or fifteen minutes, sitting in the most uncomfortable position one can possibly get into because the more pain I feel the more righteous I am. Real meditation is watching so that there is no separation between the watcher and the watched. It involves a quality of attention that has to do with seeing what is. Meditation is not a removal from the world. Real meditation is not simply a passive thing; it's an extraordinary activity, an activity without effort that involves a direct confrontation with that which is, always containing within it the eternal.

If we have been actually examining ourselves during these talks, then what we have been doing is real meditation, for real meditation is to come into direct contact with ourselves, not by looking for states that originate in thought that we may be looking for—Nirvana, Samadi. These states live in idea, desire, ambition. Real meditation is the observation of what I am, which may involve desire and ambition. Real meditation is its own blessing, its own benediction, its own end, which is actually creative living. Ordinarily what goes under the name of meditation is just another way of tranquilizing oneself, of removing oneself from the actuality of what is, of getting lost in one's desires, whether it be for eternal life or bliss (just another idea, for real bliss is very different than any idea one may have about it). So how does one meditate? Where is the path? Do you know what a path is? It's where people have been before. But there's no path. There's no way. Meditation is the blazing of the frontiers of the unknown, which is pathless.

Meditation requires seriousness, which is not a presumed seriousness, it does not negate the humor of living. It is seriousness that involves a care and attention. I must care about finding out what I am. How does one start meditating? One starts meditating by starting, by looking. The looking is the meditation, and the meditation is the movement. Yet meditation is not a thing that aims toward moving anywhere. Meditation is endless. There is nowhere to go; there just is meditation. It's a way of living, a way of living now with fantastic energy, which is being always on the crest of the unknown, which is dangerous for there is no security. But the reality of it is there is no security anywhere, and all the securities of insurance policies and the usual things we cloak ourselves with are just not real. You cannot create or buy security. There isn't any such thing.

What we've been doing here together, a human being can do quietly or in relationship. It does not take a removal from the world, although occasionally a removal from our usual environment changes one's view so that one can begin to observe oneself. A person in meditation doesn't have to be anywhere; one is always with oneself. I think this is a bit different than what we ordinarily think about when we think of meditation. You may listen to people who come from thousands of years of authority, with the tradition of centuries behind them, and they will tell you something quite different. They will tell you that meditation will lead you into a bliss, into a joy. But meditation is its own bliss, which leads nowhere. You may believe them, and it is difficult not to, because of the images they present and the traditions that we have been conditioned to accept. Or you may believe this person—but to do either is deadly; find out for yourself what meditation is about.

To be aware, alert, responsive and responsible, is to be an adult. To be totally here is to be totally in relationship. As I get to know myself I get to know that what I am is a being in relationship. Fundamentally what we are is a part of an energy system. It is awareness, a moment to moment awareness that brings a seeing of the totality and connectedness of all things. Meditation, then, is not a removal from relationship, but rather a seeing of the nature of oneself in relationship.

Much of what is called meditation promises something called ego loss. One cannot seek ego loss, for it is the ego itself that seeks ego loss for its own glorification. It's an ego trip because it involves the seeker's particular advancement, all of which is nonsense, actually. That's just another way of separation. The more people you convince you are a higher being, the more you are sure you are a higher being yourself.

Real seeing, real humility comes not from cultivation. It comes from seeing that the actuality of it is that I am really no different than you. We are not different in terms of levels, of good or better. Can my liver be better than my heart? Can my toe be better than my hand? Can I be better than you, or higher? Really?

Question. Are you saying that it isn't possible to find teachers?

Answer. That's all there are—teachers. Obviously I'm teaching. To live is to teach and to learn. To be a total human being is to be a teacher and a learner. That's what life is all about in its most creative aspects. If a teacher becomes an authority, then I'm afraid there's no teacher at all, there's just an authority. What authorities do is cut off learning totally, because you get involved in belief. What is the first thing an authority demands? Doesn't he demand belief? You have to listen to me, which means you have to believe what I tell you and suspend your own inquiry, which immediately sets up conflict and violence. Fundamentally that's what classical religions do, but it has nothing whatever to do with a religious framework of mind. A religious state of mind cannot operate in a religious system. Religion does not live in a temple; it lives only in a human being.

The game of Zen comes out of the past and its structures. Eventually, the focus of Zen is to do away with structures. You hear about stories in which the Zen master renounces his masterhood, or how Buddha fought the creation of Buddhism. If you look very carefully at it you see why. All structures, all paths, all organizations eventually destroy freedom, they ignore the unknown and stifle the living. But you have to find it out for yourself.

For centuries organizations and religions have kept us children, because we are very manageable as children and willing to give up our adulthood for our spiritual hopes and desires. We are manipulatable. Part of the whole business of "being on the path" is to run from one manipulator to another until you see yourself being manipulated, then you don't have to do it anymore.

But there is no time for it anymore. The pressures and the challenges of today do not permit endless wandering. We could blow ourselves up any minute. We're making the world more and more uninhabitable. Cosmically, it doesn't matter at all, but there is programmed into me an interest in my species.

Again, the important thing is not to agree. Agreeing doesn't matter at all. The important thing is to look at living and see for yourself what it's all about. Then you'll know, and you won't have to be told; you'll become a light unto yourself, which is what meditation is all about.

Question. How did you arrive at your definition of meditation?
Answer. I once heard a man talk, and what he said was similar to what we have been talking about. What he said struck me deeply. Although I didn't understand it in an intellectual way,

it made a deep impression on me and I began to look and as I began to look, I began to see. Then one day it happened—instantly—the whole thing just opened up and was there, the nature of thought and meditation. It just happens. It happens from looking. After the mind turns in this direction and begins to look, it is very difficult to look in other directions, because there is a directness in this way of seeing. You can find it out for yourself. Start seeing yourself.

All of the books and all of the old religious teachings, perhaps in a parenthetical phrase or a footnote, say there's only one place to look and that's within. Then they spend the rest of the time telling you to do exactly the opposite. By looking within you can find this out for yourself. To know what meditation is, is to know what thought is. To know what those meditative techniques are all about, is to know greed and the hunger of desire and all that's involved in it.

The way it is is not the way most of us want things to be. We want to be able to progress step by step from one mechanical means to another, through a system that guarantees that if we do the rituals properly then someday the doors of heaven will open for us. If one ever does get into contact with that which is eternal, with that total energy that cannot be named (which is not a function of the projections of mind, the spinning of webs of thought) one sees that it is something totally beyond structure, something that does not come from the asking for it. It is something that is totally different and beyond all the imaginations of mind, which is why mind can never get you there. All one can do is open the window, then the breeze may blow in. What meditation is, is the opening of the window to the seeing of oneself—totally.

How does one look? I have been asked if the looking is not again another desire, getting caught up in the old game again. It is not. The looking is looking. It's not trying to look. It doesn't involve effort.

Meditation does not involve practice, for practice is mechanical. Nor does it involve effort, for effort always removes you from what is. If my mind is busy and I am noisy, then that is what is.

To see it so there is no space between the seer and the seen is meditation. The seeing that I am the noise contains a movement, an energy without force or effort.

What is called "enlightenment" is not a marketable commodity. People don't want it. What people want are their ideas of pleasure, what they think the world should be. Enlightenment as a state or a possession is just an idea. If I call myself enlightened I am talking about the past: I am in memory and out of memory I build an image of myself. As soon as I have an image of myself as an enlightened being or anything else, I have removed myself from growth. I have shadowed the living moment. The eternal is just here. It's the moment. Here and now. The reason I don't see it is that I don't look—it's really quite simple. Meditation is a way of looking, a turn of mind that just looks and does not ask. One of the things that it can look at is the fact that I am always asking. I cannot make that go away either, but I can begin to observe the nature of asking. That, too, is meditation.

Question. You say meditation takes no effort. To me that implies passivity and stagnation. Looking at my life, it seems that any time I moved into something new great effort was required.

Answer. There are times when one moves into something new and great effort appears to be involved. If one looks clearly at this it is not the movement into the new that takes effort, but rather hanging on to the residue of the old. The old pleasures, securities, fears, make demands that bind one in conflict. It is here that effort lies.

Of course the inquiry here takes a great deal of energy. I think that many of us equate energy with effort, but they are not the same. Have you ever watched children play? There is an enormous energy there, enormous attention, but no effort. No one is forcing the child to play, not even the child itself. What we have been talking about has got to be like play, which means you must be really interested in yourself and how you work. Real interest contains passion, which is effortless. In fact, our efforts are designed to control passion, out of fear.

It takes no effort to see "what is." Say I put you in a room and in the center of the room is a flower on a table. In the flower

I put a sensing device to record when you look at the flower. I tell you that if you can stay in the room for a month and not look at the flower, I'll give you one million dollars, enlightenment, or whatever you want. How much effort will you have to spend not to see the flower? It's there; in order not to see it you must be constantly on guard. So, too, it takes great effort, great guardedness not to see ourselves.

We fear that if we give up effort, stop trying, we will vegetate and become dull. Yet it is the effort itself that is always reaching for ideas (that come out of conditioning) which keeps us from the new. If one is in touch with what is, it is not possible to stagnate. For "what is" is always new, fresh; and if one is responsible to the new, that response-ability is the creative aspect of life. Real meditation is not a removal from life, but life as creation.

CHAPTER 12

EVOLUTION

At first blush it may appear that our inquiry is itself rather self-centered. Turning inward could probably be viewed as an escape from external turmoil. Actually, however, the inner and outer are not different. The turmoil of the world is just an expression of the inner confusion of people. People create the world in their own image; if the world is confused, self-centered, violent, falling apart, it's because I am—because we are.

Let's look at why meditation and awareness in these times have such tremendous urgency for each individual and for the species itself.

We live in a time of great turmoil, with enormous problems. There are the problems of ecology involving the fact that we are making the world uninhabitable, the problems of cities, racial tensions, alcohol and other drugs, the economic problems of distributing goods in an increasingly automated world where wealth tends to polarize, the problems of loneliness and sorrow. So many problems seem almost insurmountable.

We treat our problems in an isolated way, trying to solve them independently of one another. We create committees, rehabilitation centers, departments, yet the problems increase. We feel helpless, for what can a person do?

The fabric of our society is breaking down and trying to solve these problems from within the old structures that compartmentalize them only feeds the confusion. The problems mentioned are only symptoms. If only the symptoms are dealt with, the sickness pops out some other place. The real problem is that the old ways no longer work.

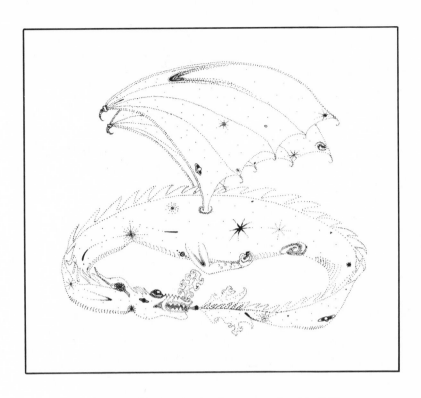

Memry the Dragon is always creating his Self

Many people worrying about the problem of drugs are trying to do something about it. The fact is that destructive drugs (I do not use the term destructive evaluatively, but physiologically) are in the grade schools, not only in so-called slum areas, but in all areas. In the vain hope of trying to solve this problem, we outlaw drugs, build rehabilitation centers, do this and that—but we are not looking at the real problem at all.

The problem of drugs is not drugs. The problem is that they offer some people a more interesting alternative than living life. And so long as that is the case there will be a continuing problem with drugs. For example, heroin is extraordinarily dulling. The problem with heroin is that people really want to be dulled away from living and that is not only the problem of such drugs. It's the problem of living today. The use of drugs will actually increase unless there's a change in the structure of living. You can outlaw drugs, but you cannot do away with them. You cannot merely treat symptoms and expect a deep cure. You can try, but it doesn't work. Much of the old order is breaking down—that seems to be the real problem.

Living is challenge and response, and problems are challenges. What responses are appropriate? What can I do? I'm just a drop in a huge ocean. How can I respond to all this and even if I do, what difference will it make? Is it possible to be truly responsible, response-able? To help us examine these questions, let us go into the nature and workings of evolution.

Are you familiar with the evolutionary mechanism and how it works? The mechanism has to do with a so-called random mutation in the reproductive tissue itself, and when changes occur in environmental pressures, the appropriate mutation is picked out and survives—the so-called "survival of the fittest."

An animal has evolved that is so clever it can change its environment and is no longer subject to the same kind of environmental evolutionary pressures. The old way of changing is no longer applicable. Yet I know there is only change or the alternative—become an evolutionary dead end and go the way of the dinosaur. The real challenge of the times is really quite simple—it's a question of survival—whether or not we as a species are going to continue to grow, change, and evolve—or not.

Have you ever asked where inside of you the mechanism for evolution lives? How does it display itself in you? What is the phenomenological impact of it, the feel of it, the way it expresses itself in living? For surely if there is such a thing as evolution, I am a product and carrier of it.

Most of us are conditioned to accept outside authorities and secondhand sources for our "knowledge." That is the way we are taught. We read about evolution in the schools and are shown external evidence of it in pictures, bones, fossils. It's intellectually fashionable to believe in evolution, and, in fact, should one not do so today, there would be ridicule. If there is such a process as evolution, then obviously I am the end result of eons of it; each of us is. Also quite obviously evolution must be passed on through me, so the mechanisms of evolution must live somewhere in me. Is it possible to get in touch with this mechanism from the inside? Not intellectually, but as a living thing. If I observe myself clearly, I find that this mechanism is the product of thousands of years of conditioning; it is programmed into me genetically. The feel of it is violence.

Violence is the internal expression of the mechanism. One way it expresses itself is in competition, which is violence. We don't look at this clearly because we don't like to look at ourselves that way, but it's there—the survival of the fittest. I compete for biomass, for food, for territory, with other species—and that is violence. I am an extraordinarily violent animal and an extraordinarily successful one. I have casually destroyed entire species around me, completely, and more are dying. I have spread my seed over the land, and as I do so other species die out. Violence is what made me successful. The violence is me; it's programmed into me.

My evolutionary advantage is my mind and brain. That's what has made our species the successful animal it is. The tiger has its claw, we have thought. I certainly can't beat up the tiger in a fight, but I can shoot him, which means I can invent guns, which come from thought. As we saw, thought is competitive, comparative, violent. I have used this tool with extraordinary success. I am king of the planet. No other species threatens me at all. As I have conquered the physical frontiers of the planet, the outlets for violence have narrowed. I have fewer of the usual external outlets for violence, so where do I direct it? It's quite obvious: I turn it on myself and the planet I live on. That's what's happening: we're destroying ourselves. That's what we are seeing today: the young against the old, black against white, this country against that, my religion against yours, male against female, female against male. These all function out of beliefs, and beliefs as we saw are themselves violent.

We are destroying the planet (the ecological problem), which, really, is just another manifestation of violence. Out of my cleverness, I've created weapons for destroying myself completely. We are that clever. Yet as a species we are quite adolescent. Adolescence within the species is marked by extreme self-centeredness and by the utilization of power and manipulation for their own sakes. That describes us as a species: we have extraordinary power that adolescents are not capable of handling.

If we as a species are to become adults, we must come to terms with our violence. The challenge of the times is actually evolutionary: are we as a species going to move into adulthood? The old evolutionary mechanism, the old way that change has come about, is no longer working, for it's based on violence and that violence conditioned into me over the centuries has turned on itself. Many of us have been intellectually conditioned to believe that violence doesn't work. Religions and societies have preached nonviolence while engaging in the very violence they condemn—religious and social wars, missionaries destroying cultures, inquisitions and other pressures to conform. This is our history. The simple fact is that violence does work very well, or rather it did work very well. The challenge of our times is that it's no longer working; we've become too good at it.

Is it possible for there to be a new mechanism of change that's not violent? Please keep in mind that this person is not saying that violence is wrong or bad. Also, I am not suggesting here that violence was not appropriate in times past for the evolution and survival of the species; via the old mechanism our seed has spread with abundance, which has now also become a problem. Rather, what I'm doing here is simply looking at violence and how it works.

The structures of society are not working, but there's no such thing as society apart from the people who create it. We create society in our own image. If society is violent, confused, self-centered, it's simply because I am, because you are. The old evolutionary mechanism, which is genetically programmed into me, is no longer appropriate; my conditioning, which is what I am, is now working against me. A species that turns its violence on itself as we are, is heading for self-destruction. What am I to do?

What we have been discussing in these talks is actually an evolution of the very mechanism of evolution itself that can bring about a real mutation in the cellular structure, such that the change is not a function of the old mechanism but of the new one—a new evolutionary principle. Is this possible? It seems so remote from everything we've learned. Can the mechanism of change itself change? Ordinarily we think of the mind and the body as different, yet we're aware of some connection. If you take a drink of alcohol or sample another psychotropic drug, something mechanical is done to the body. Psychological change, a change in awareness, accompanies the physical change. We tend to think of this as a one-way door, but actually it is not, for if awareness changes there is also necessarily a physiological change. Actually, the mind and the body are not separate. They are just different aspects of one energy system.

For there to be a total change in awareness there is automatically a change in the very cellular structure itself—a mutation therefore both of brain and mind. The old mechanism predicated on violence has lived largely unconsciously in us. Just as the time for adolescence is past, so too is the time of unconscious evolution past if we are to survive. When one is young and cared for, there's a reluctance to move into adulthood for youth has its beauty and carefreeness. One can observe a resistance to moving into adulthood within the species. Most human beings remain children content to play at being adult. It's not surprising that one can observe a similar resistance and growing pains in the species itself. Yet the planet is crying for a caretaker—a species that takes care. It can occur only if we move beyond violence, for violence is totally self-centered. Violence is a great pleasure. Look at your anger—not your judgments about your anger—but your anger itself. What an enormous pleasure it is, and how we cultivate it and use it for release.

Living is challenge and response, and we as a species are facing the challenge of evolution, which has to do with a new principle of change. How does it happen? If I try to make it happen I can only try to do so out of my old conditioning, which does not bring forth the new, therefore, conflict. I feel the urgency of change in me, but any changing I try to do through effort only creates more conflict, more violence. I could try to cultivate nonviolence, but the cultivation of nonviolence is only another form of violence. What am I to do?

To see the nature of my conditioning (genetic as well as social) which includes seeing how change occurred in the past, to see the violence in it—to see it, not to judge it—to see how it's no longer appropriate to survival, to see all of this is to move. If you see the danger of a tree falling on you, then you move from it. The seeing is the movement; there is no gap, no space, no time between the seeing and the movement. You don't know which way you are going to jump, and where you find yourself is always a surprise. Similarly, if you see the danger of the old way of being, even though it was programmed into you, then the seeing is a movement and the movement is change, and the change is a mutation of mind—a real revolution. For the nature of my conditioning, including my genetic conditioning, is as dangerous to me and the species as a tree falling. As a species the tree is falling on us. Movement, change, evolution only come with the total seeing of this—the seeing that is total awareness is the new mechanism that moves beyond our unconscious conditionings into the conscious. Meditation is the key to this, for it is in meditation that seeing comes. Seeing generates movement; actually the seeing and the movement are one.

The old order is breaking down and many people are talking revolution. By revolution some of them mean using force and violence to tear down the old order and install a new one, which is the way so-called changes have occurred through the centuries. The new order then becomes the oppressor followed by another revolution. That is the old way; it's endless because external revolution brings no fundamental change. The power and the distribution of goods may change, so that instead of people with suits and crewcuts having the power, perhaps people with long hair and beards will; it really doesn't matter, it's the same thing under a different guise. The only real change is for a human being to change; the only real revolution is within one's self. It's all very personal.

If I come to terms with the nature of myself, including my violence, if I see its danger then change occurs. If one person changes, it's a real thing. It's only by human change that any kind of change occurs. When human beings see for themselves the real danger to survival in the old way of being, the seeing is the movement. There are no authorities, no experts, nobody to do it for you. To go to an authority is to go to someone whose authority comes from the past. It's the past as it lives in memory that has brought us here. There is no one who can tell you what to do. There will, of course, be people who will be glad to do so, but they are minions of the old, of the known.

The challenge of the times is whether the human race will survive. In order for the response to be adequate, there can be no authorities. To be adequate the response must be new, creative, not out of the known. There are no authorities, there is only you and me; that may be a frightening thing. But for one human being to change, really change, it's like dropping a stone in a pond: there are ripples and these ripples affect others. That is the way change occurs—personally—from person to person. Not from institution to institution, not from leader to disciple, but from person to person. It's all very individual and personal.

What we have been talking about is a revolution of mind, an internal change that is not achieved through asking for it. You don't know what to ask for. How do you ask for something you don't know? The change only occurs through revelation and by that I don't mean anything mystical, esoteric, or out of the ken of ordinary people. By revelation I mean something quite simple: revelation is seeing—an immediacy that does not occur in time or in thought. It occurs instantly—whether the instant is a second or a year doesn't matter. Seeing is revelation, the only real revolution there is, and it is the only way I can totally respond to any real challenge. The response must be new, if it is to be adequate. The nature of any challenge is that it is new. If it were simply a repeated event, it would be no real challenge. The creative aspects of living involve meeting challenges freshly, not simply out of the past.

We have asked, "Why bother to be interested in awareness at all? It's so self-centered." But it is only if the self, the human being, individually, comes to terms with him- or herself that real change occurs. We are living in extraordinarily challenging times; never before have the challenges of life occurred as they are now, so there is no one who can give you an answer. Many people want to be experts and if you go to the experts they will tell you to do this or that—let's go back to the Bible, or the Gita, or the Upanishads, or whatever. Let's go *back* because the old masters have all the wisdom. Or let's follow this leader or that. I'm afraid if we do that we're lost. All of the old structures have gotten us exactly where we are now.

The challenges are not met out of the past. They are only met from creativity, which means newness, which means responsibility, which means seeing. Action that is creative, that is not bound by conflict which creates the dross of guilt and regret, comes only from a total seeing. The seeing is the movement.

We like to give the responsibility to the authorities and have the experts tell us what to do. But as we have seen there are no experts; there is no authority; there is just you. The giving of one's responsibility to someone else is very strange indeed, because responsibility really means response-ability, the ability to respond adequately, which can never be given away.

Again, it is important neither to agree nor disagree, nor to try to formulate this into a pleasant or convenient or familiar structure that one can comfortably operate with. The important thing is to begin to look at the way one actually works, and to look at oneself is to look at oneself in relationship to the whole world. The inner and the outer are not different. For me to change, so too the world changes. For me not to change, the world will not. That's just the way of it. For one human being to become aware is to have the spark spread. It touches; it makes a difference.

Ordinarily awareness is not a marketable item at all. People don't want it. Civilization certainly doesn't want it. Society has no use for it at all. Awareness is a wild thing, not a tame beast; it is not respectable, which means of course it doesn't respond to the usual pushing of buttons of conditioning that are used to control us. There is then great pressure not to see.

It seems awareness only emerges when there is a tremendous urgency, so that change is necessary. And that's what's happening now. The world is crying out for movement because the old ways are not working. Awareness is necessary because it means confrontation with the new. It's frightening and dangerous, but living is dangerous; you can walk out in the street and be hit by a car.

What am I to do? I see the urgency of change, but any time I try to change myself, whether it's through a technique, or a master, guru, school of philosophy, psychology, or whatever, I'm always involved in the old because to change myself is an effort, which means conflict. I have an idea that I should be something else, so I feel there's a gap between the "is" and the "ought." I feel the urgency in me and I want to move. The idea of movement contains within it a conflict, because all I can do is move to the old. You can only seek what you know—you cannot seek the unknown. So how do I go about it? The very process of seeking, which necessarily brings about fear, through ambition, is the bind.

In looking at oneself, in looking at the problems one faces, what we ordinarily want to do is eliminate the problems and find ultimate solutions so that all our problems are solved. But that's really just another product of thought. To live creatively is always to live with challenge, always to live with problems. The problems really aren't the problem. The problem is that our responses are inadequate, incomplete. There is an interesting way of recognizing for yourself whether the response to a challenge has been adequate. When the challenge isn't met creatively, then something happens. The challenge lives in memory. You go over it. I should have done this, I should have done that. It stays with you. But when a response is adequately met, it's gone. You can leave it. You can die to it, then move on to the next problem.

Ideas keep you away from direct contact with the living thing, which is never captured by thought, ideas, or structures. A living tree, a human being, a moment of extraordinary intensity cannot be captured by symbol. Yet this is how we live, trying to recapture. We want answers, but as soon as something is answered, it's past and gone. Real learning, which is not the mere accumulation of knowledge, is not answers—it's questions. When you put the right question to yourself at the right time, the answer is often contained within the question. If you can see the problem clearly enough to pin it in a question, you also can see the only possible move for you.

In general what we do is take our past successes and try to apply them to new things; here habit forms and creativity leaves. As we get older and older we become more knowledgeable, which means that we have more habits. The older we get and the more knowledge we have about the world, the more difficult it is to live in newness, in freshness. The more we hunger for the memories of love as we get older, the more it seems to slip by us. The spark, the thing we hold in memory just doesn't seem to be the way it used to be.

If life is secure and the pleasures of living come easily, then there isn't much interest in awareness, and we get easily caught in the habits and the conditionings of living that get piled up as we get older. In this day and age it's very difficult for one to remain in one's habitual modes. The challenges of the times are great; ignoring them creates extraordinary conflict. Our structures as they carry us along are actually built by us; they are just a manifestation of what we are. As these structures seem to be inappropriate, it becomes more difficult to maintain one's habits and the securities we strive for. If the structures are to change and become appropriate for the pressures and needs of a changing world, we must change. Is it possible for a human being actually to come to terms with the reality of what he or she is, and in doing so, for there to be a newness, a creativity, that is not just a function of the old patterns?

We are on an evolutionary crest and whether we will or will not respond to that challenge remains to be seen. The response to the challenge cannot be done for us by anyone else. No one is going to tell you how to go about doing it for the simple reason that it's new to everyone. It's not a matter for experts or authorities or gurus. It's a personal matter for every human being in confrontation with himself.

We have the idea that what peace or bliss is, is a life with no problems, a life of staid equilibrium where nothing affects one. But that isn't peace or bliss, it's merely an idea. Peace or bliss is not a cessation of problems, but the ability to respond to problems in an unfettered, unconflicted, creative way, so that total energy is involved. And the question is, of course, whether a human being can confront himself so that the challenges or problems can be met and dealt with creatively.

Real creativity only comes about through a quieting of the old. That's what meditation is all about. It is not passive, not a removal, or withdrawal from the world. Real meditation is a way of living, a way of seeing the world, because that's all there actually is—being in the world.

Question. It seems to me that religions have been trying to bring about nonviolence in people, and in myself I have worked at destroying my violence, yet as you say, violence is still here. You make me feel hopeless. There seems to be nothing I can do.

Answer. First, the feeling of hopelessness involves what we've been looking at: wanting things to be other than what they are and fearful they will not be. That is not being hopeless; it is only when one is truly hope-less that one can see what is.

Religions, structures, societies, people have all tried to cultivate nonviolence, but the attempt at cultivating nonviolence is itself violent. I have ideas, beliefs, which as we saw bring forth violence, that I should not be violent, that violence is bad. So through force or effort (violence again) I try to destroy my violence. The whole process is violence. Violence only leaves when one sees its inappropriateness, then it leaves without force, without effort.

Question. You seem to be saying that there should be a revolution of mind. That the human race should evolve. Isn't that ambition?

Answer. From a cosmic point of view it does not matter a bit if humanity survives or not. Everything passes. The dinosaur did, and human beings may, too. Yet there is programmed into me an interest in seeing whether the particular form that I am an example of has, in fact, completed its dance. Actually, we as a species are quite young, and we are now in the growing pains of losing our youth and becoming adults. There is no guarantee it will happen. In fact, I haven't said we should evolve. What I have said is that if we are to grow, and meeting challenges is growth, then a mutation, an evolution is necessary. There is no ambition or evaluation here, simply description.

Question. You have said that thought is never new, but you have also said that thought invents guns. The invention of guns has made an enormous impact on the world and has really seemed to change things. So here it appears that thought did bring newness.

Answer. In the realms of the purely mechanical, thought, through recombining the old, the known, occasionally does come up with seemingly new ways of channeling energy, which is what a gun is.

But even here the actual seeing of a new way to channel energy, though coming from thought, is not thought itself. There is always a leap from thought. Insights which are *sights in* are not done by thought but only occur in an instant when thought stops. Did the invention of guns actually bring newness? If by *newness* one means a change in the forms that structures take, then obviously the invention of guns has done that. But if by newness one is referring to an alteration of the very structure itself then just as obviously guns have not changed this. Guns have just allowed me to express my violence in another way. Real change is not disguising the old in another form.

In the nonmechanical aspects of living which involve total relationship, the limitations of thought, which we have been examining, are more obvious. Yet even here, as we saw, thought has its place as a practical tool. Living relationship ceases when the tool becomes the master.

Question. Violence has always been with us. Why is it not appropriate if channeled properly?

Answer. Who is going to channel it properly and is not the channeling itself violent? There was a time when we were relatively isolated from one another in that what we did and how we lived our lives didn't affect many others outside the immediate family or village. Now the world is a village; technology has made the feedbacks and communications of the world immediate and global. When Japan pollutes the ocean, it's my ocean too. When the United States tests an atomic bomb and fills the air with radiation, it's everyone's atmosphere. Since people are interconnected around the world, what we do has great effect. So if we are to move into adulthood, it is necessary for each of us to be truly responsible to the whole world. Out of our old violent modes of conditioning we still treat the rest of the world as other, as separate from us. It is this self-centered activity that is no longer appropriate.

Some people want to turn back to the old, simple ways of living. There is no turning back. Only advanced technology can feed the billions of people, but technology need not be destructive. It is destructive only because people are.

Question. I have always thought that one learns through experience, then by remembering one's past experiences fewer mistakes are made. One of the things I'm getting here is a negation of experience. If we were to negate our experience, either our personal experience or accumulated experience of history (what I believe you call conditioning) then I do not see how we would ever have moved from the caves.

Answer. It is important to see that this person is not talking about negating the past, or memory, or one's conditioning. How can you do that? If one tries to negate the past, is there not a negator who is trying to shut something out? We cannot run away from our conditioning; we are our conditioning. Creative or new movement does not come by negating the old but rather it moves from it. Negation is simply reaction that contains in it the very thing being reacted against. To see the inappropriateness of our conditioning, of the evolutionary mechanism that lives in us, is not to react against it or negate it. To see totally one's violence, how it separates you from me, to see the pleasure in it and the sorrow—the seeing is the movement.

The movement out of one's conditioning is the revolution of mind and is the thrust of evolution itself. This person does realize that what he is talking about is very different from the way we ordinarily think of evolution. Ordinarily we think of it as an unconscious process following its own mysterious routes. What we have been discussing is a new evolutionary mechanism that is based upon consciousness, awareness. A change in awareness necessarily involves a change in the cells themselves. That is what evolution is actually all about—changes in awareness.

Question. What do you mean by "violence"?

Answer. Violence is fragmenting the world into the internal and external and treating the external as "other," as "not me." We do this even within ourselves. Many of us call ourselves our minds and relegate our bodies to secondary status. That too is violence. I realize this is a different way of looking at violence than we ordinarily do. Only by looking within yourself will you ever find out if the roots of violence lie in fragmentation.

Question. What do you see we need to do in order to meet the challenges? If we cannot *try* to change, what then?

Answer. If we are to survive as a species, responsibility is needed, which, of course, means reaching adulthood as a race. Growth is not the mere accumulation of experience; one only grows when one moves, and to move one must leave old ways behind. Not through negation, but rather through a total seeing does real growth occur. Growth may be painful because there are many pleasures of childhood that one is loath to give up. You can see this in your own movement from what we call adolescence to what is considered adulthood. So it is with us as a species: We are undergoing growing pains. There is no truly responsible species on the planet today. Yet the energies that are now in play cannot be handled by children; the energies are too powerful. That is the challenge you and I face. No one will do it for you and to wait for someone else is to remain a child. Real meditation is the key that unlocks the door to the unknown. Real meditation is the key to a whole new process of evolution: an evolution of the very mechanism of evolution. Why should the mechanism itself not be part of the process of total movement, a movement from the unconscious to the aware? The old mechanism was based on unconscious processes, which by their very unconscious nature control us and keep us children. A movement in the mechanism from unconscious to conscious is a movement into adulthood, and the real question is whether we as a species are going to grow up.

Question. If what you say is true, then we are doomed. Humanity as a whole will not see this.

Answer. The question is not, "Is everybody going to do it?" The question is, "Am I going to?" If only a small percent of the planet— ten thousand people, one thousand, or even one hundred—were to see the challenge, and move with it, the energy would be remarkable and would spread. It is not the desire to evolve that brings evolution, but rather the total seeing of oneself. Total seeing is what meditation is all about.